IMPROVE YOUR MARATHON AND HALF MARATHON RUNNING

David Chalfen

Foreword by Bud Baldaro

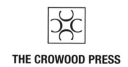

THE CROWOOD PRESS

First published in 2012 by
The Crowood Press Ltd
Ramsbury, Marlborough
Wiltshire SN8 2HR

www.crowood.com

British Library Cataloguing-in-Publication Data
A catalogue record for this book is available from the British Library.

ISBN 978 1 84797 390 0

Typeset by Jean Cussons Typesetting, Diss, Norfolk

Printed and bound in India by Replika Press Pvt Ltd

CONTENTS

CONTENTS

FOREWORD

David Chalfen is wonderfully well placed to write a book on marathon and half-marathon training. I have known Dave for many years and in that time have never failed to be impressed by his thirst for knowledge of a sport he loves profoundly.

As a coach for many years at club, student and area/international level, Dave certainly 'knows his stuff'. He has been a student of the sport for numerous years and is a true aficionado of the road scene. Passionate and inspired by runners of all ability levels, he brings to the table a life-long love of the sport combined with a depth of knowledge and the ability to develop his points in a rational, accessible and comprehensible manner. He possesses a genuine insight into both the needs of runners and their patient progression, plus of course the very specific demands of the events.

Well planned and well written, this addition to the lore of road running will add significantly to required reading. The book is refreshingly honest and realistic, conveying well Dave's desire to see runners of all levels realize their full potential. I have no doubt that many runners and coaches will benefit tremendously from Dave's keenness and passion and above all the directness of his knowledge, so well presented in this book.

This book makes for happy and stimulating reading – ensure that you put into practice these good ideas.

Bud Baldaro
Former UK Athletics Marathon coach and personal coach to Hannah England, World Championships Silver medallist in 2011 and to many British international runners

To Rosa, a most wonderful daughter.

ABOUT THE AUTHOR

David Chalfen has been coaching endurance running for over a decade and has been running for more than thirty years. He is a Level 4 Performance UKA Coach and is an Area Endurance Coach Mentor for England Athletics, developing the endurance coaching network in North London and Hertfordshire. He has coached numerous distance runners ranging from national level to modest club level, and operates both as a volunteer coach – as a member of Serpentine Running Club – and via a website www.runcoach1to1.com. He has also acted as Team Manager for various international athletes at major marathons in Europe and Asia and has written feature articles about endurance running for Athletics Weekly. He competed at County level and ran ten marathons under 2 hours 35 minutes, with a best of 2.32. He lives in London. He was educated in North London and at Oxford University. This is his first book.

PREFACE

I was sitting in an Internet café in the hills in Andalucia when I received the email equivalent of a cold call from Crowood inviting me to write this book. My first reaction was one of suspicion akin to receiving an email from a West African 'bank' enquiring after my mother's maiden name and asking to verify my Internet banking password. But it was bona fide and many thanks to Crowood editor Hannah Shakespeare for her faith in adding my name to the endurance writing publications list.

At the risk of self-aggrandisement, or perhaps just showing that I'm an embarrassingly slow learner, the knowledge and experience that has gone into this book has been almost forty years in the making. The first seeds were sown in 1972 when as a very shy eight-year-old I watched the 1972 Olympics from Munich. Amidst the British highlights and the deadly intrusion of the terrorist attacks on the Israeli team, it was the long-distance races that stuck in my mind. Finnish legend Lasse Virén achieving the 5,000m and 10,000m double on the track, and the wiry USA runner Frank Shorter coming home for a dominant marathon win had a key role in triggering the growth of long-distance running in the Western world. I thought it looked very exciting and wanted to be part of it. And so started my fascination with long-distance running.

By a mixture of luck and design, this brought me into some hotbeds of endurance running. My very first tentative track sessions at Shaftesbury Harriers in north-west London were done with one lane kept aside whilst the then World Record Holder for 10,000m, Dave Bedford, went through sessions trying to recapture his 1973 glory days. I progressed and was able to wear the Barnet Schools vest with some pride but little competence.

Through my later teens I persisted with a stable level of mediocrity. The typical scenario was that if I beat another Under 17 or Under 20 athlete they would see retirement from the sport – and in a couple of extreme cases emigrating to South America with an entirely new identity – as the only logical option to preserve some vestiges of self-respect. At University I could just about describe future World Cup Marathon Champion and 2.08 marathon performer Richard Nerurkar as a training partner on those days when his recovery run and my threshold effort happened to coincide.

To show how the marathon world has changed, I ran my first marathon just before turning eighteen. In an event that wasn't even classified as an official competitive event, I placed forty-second in a time of 2hr 42min. Thirty years on, there is no race in Britain outside the mighty London Marathon where this sort of time would place so relatively far down the field.

Typical of many coaches, it was only after stopping my own competitive running (well, as competitive as my short stumpy legs and overzealous engagement with Mr Kipling's exceedingly good cakes could manage) that I acquired the objectivity to drill down into the details of how to really optimize one's endurance-running ability, whatever level that ability is. It's a cliché that is only partly true, but distance running is in many ways the easiest sport to do – just put on your kit, head out the door and run, sometimes hard and sometimes easy, and if you do this very regularly you will improve considerably. However, it's also just as easy to become a regularly injured runner or an underachieving runner. Indeed, most experienced runners will at different stages encounter both situations and the goal – which I hope this book will contribute to – is to ensure that the large majority of one's running years are spent achieving the best results that are achievable for each individual's ability and training commitment.

My time so far in coaching has been supported by all of the following who contrib-ute to the immense enjoyment we gain from the fulfilling yet existentially futile attempts to help people run a long way a little bit quicker than the last time they tried it:

In particular, Bud Baldaro and Geoff Williams, great motivators and special people who have such a lasting and positive influence on so many. And they also help them to run faster. Outside the running world, Kevin Hickey MBE has been a tremendously wise and supportive mentor and adviser on the broader aspects of sports coaching.

Also my friend and clubmate Urban Bettag, a master of constructive criticism. And Bev Kitching; Stella Bandu; Dave Newport; Martin Rush; Peter McHugh; Nick Anderson; Dave Sunderland; Bryan Smith; and Ian Ladbrooke.

Photo credits – Urban Bettag, Ian Hodge and Rosa Chalfen.

CHAPTER 1

INTRODUCTION

Who Is This Book For?

Here is an outline of what this book offers:

- A guide to the training principles of both distances that explains what is contained within the training plans.
- Some detailed programmes that show how the principles can be addressed on a practical level and evolved as the runner's experience – and hopefully also their commitment and performance – evolves.
- Some case histories of runners with high levels of commitment and modest levels of talent to show what can be done – a combination of information and inspiration.

The book thoroughly covers what an experienced long-distance running coach can bring to improving runners. A coach will have some grounding in: anatomy; physiology; nutrition; hydration; psychology; strength and conditioning; mentoring; and other relevant elements – but won't usually be a professionally qualified expert in all of these fields. But no apologies for that – coaches are serial magpies, dipping into anywhere they can find the extra 'one percenters' to help the people they coach.

What cannot be provided in these pages are any guarantees as to how successful your running will be, even if you follow all the advice. Nor does the content address beyond a relevant level of theoretical and practical detail the full minutiae of some of the sports science that has informed and guided the training principles and programmes. Therefore, you will find that the book has a relatively large proportion of its pages allocated to the 'bread and butter' of training for endurance running. There is a lesser emphasis on aspects such as nutrition and sports medicine, because there are publications available by proven experts in these fields.

This approach is also intended to give the book a greater 'added value' to what you can find on the Internet. There is vast information on the web regarding diet, physiology, static stretching and race calendars, and there is perhaps limited benefit in simply replicating this data in book form. What this book does is to offer a logical and detailed approach on how to plan and carry out your endurance training and racing, underpinned by the other factors that will affect your performance. Readers are then signposted to other specialist publications if they wish to drill down into these supplementary elements. It is, as it were, the published version of how running coaches work in real life.

The running world is hugely diverse in what the profiles of 'improvers' will be. A debut marathoner may have no running background, but years of training in sports such as cycling, swimming, rowing or skiing, so although their running history may be close to zero, their aerobic base will be high. It may be much higher than someone who has been running for three years from scratch and has covered a few thousand miles in that period.

Whatever you may have seen elsewhere, this book does not categorize any of the training plans by target time. The reasoning is that some people have high levels of running talent, while other people's genetics are less naturally honed for distance running. A purported sub-3-hour marathon schedule may be followed by someone with great genes and help them do sub-2.35. Conversely, someone with much poorer endurance traits may do the same plan and struggle to break 3.30.

Of course, in addition to the genetics, there are the significant effects of gender, age and bodyweight. Specifically on gender, female performances of equal merit to men's are about 15 per cent slower. If you do the maths, you may be slightly surprised and perceive this as being harsh on assessing women's performances, but it actually reflects the fact that there are still more men than women who compete in distance races and – looking across the generality of runners – that more men become involved in serious running training.

That said, the author strongly believes that the large majority of long-distance runners, both men and women, do not realize what they can achieve and tend to overestimate what level of ability is needed to run what are pretty modest times. Of course, you have to put the work in to do so, but the challenge is in many ways the attraction.

However, let's put a few numbers onto the generalizations, to indicate what sort of runner should find this book relevant:

- You are already running regularly for much of the year and currently, or very soon, can regularly commit four days per week to some running training.
- You have already done one or more running race of at least 5km or 10km, so even if you have not yet tackled a marathon or half-marathon you are an improving runner.
- You expect to be able to run or jog all the way in your target races.

The United Kingdom rankings show that in 2010 some 1,800 men broke 3 hours for the marathon, with just under 2,000 women running sub-3.45. In the same year, 1,800 men broke 80 minutes for the half-marathon and 1,300 women dipped under 94 minutes for the distance. Within these numbers, and particularly at the lower end of these rankings, would be many veterans in their forties and occasionally a talented and committed fifty-plus athlete.

It is likely that if you can consistently follow any of the training programmes described in this book for at least a couple of years, and you are under forty-five years old and keep your Body Mass Index (BMI) at around twenty-five or lower, you should be able to get to within about 5 per cent of the times stated above as the minimum performances to make these rankings lists (see www.thepowerof10.info/rankings for full information).

The training schedules shown in later chapters are based around these premises. They are not intended to be for 'Get Me Round' runners, nor in all likelihood would one expect a national level runner – say Top Twenty or so in the UK rankings – to be tapping into this book, as the author would hope that at that level of ability and commitment there is an individual coach–athlete relationship to optimize the runner's talent. The schedules can be used by anybody between these two categories.

Indeed, if you progress from the schedules provided here, follow the advice on how to move to the next stage, then use the details from the advanced runners' case histories as illustrations of how to really stretch yourself, there is no reason why this book could not be used to guide you towards marathon times heading towards 2.30 for men and 2.50 for women. That level of commitment will not be for everyone and will take a few years rather than a few months, but the option is there if that is something you would like to prioritize.

The training details are divided into different levels and the author suggests that – irrespective of your current Personal Bests (PBs) – if you wish to structure your training around any of these programmes, you start with whatever level looks like the most gradual step forwards from the current volume and intensity at which you are working.

Whatever information you may gain from this book, the one thing it will not do is put on your running kit and get you out of the door for a training run. Or as legendary American basketball coach John Wooden put it, 'Do not let what you cannot do interfere with what you can do.'

Enjoy the read and good luck with your running performances.

The Marathon and Half-Marathon Race Distances

As an introduction to why this book is focused on the marathon and half-marathon rather than entitled, say, *Improving at 11 and 22 Miles*, here is a very brief history lesson. The marathon was used as the long-distance race in the modern Olympics when they were introduced in 1896 in Athens, to recreate the outline of the track and field programme in the Ancient Greek Olympics. In a bow to nineteenth-century etiquette, athletes wore

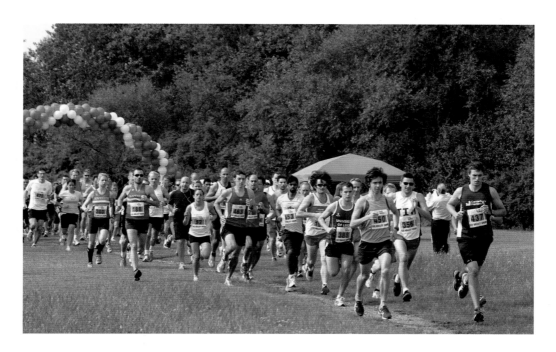

Most races now attract a wide range of running experience and performance.

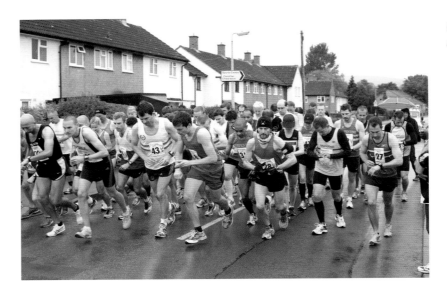

*Old-style, low-key
road-race start.*

clothes rather than competing nude as they had in ancient days.

In the early days, distances varied around 25 miles (40km). For the 1908 Games in London, however, the course was extended to ensure that athletes finished in front of the Royal Box, occupied by Queen Alexandra. The distance that day turned out to be 26 miles 385yd (42.195km). Further variations on the theme followed until from 1921 onwards, when the World Athletics Federation came into being, the distance was agreed as 42.195km. As a globally recognizable word, the marathon distance seems likely to be with us for as long as people seek long-distance running challenges. So should you ever find the last few miles of a marathon particularly hellish (reading to the end of this book is intended to make this a less likely occurrence), then you can blame the Royal Family with historical accuracy on your side.

For any runners with an element of competitive spirit, there is a very fundamental challenge of wishing to see if they can run a long way without stopping; and then to see if they can cover the distance faster than other people and faster than their previous attempts.

In Britain, until the very late 1970s, the road-race options below marathon focused on 5-, 10- and 20-milers, particularly 10s, whilst in Europe it was mainly 10, and 20 or 25km. As the marathon boom in Britain – which took place about three or four years after a similar trend in the USA – caused a huge upsurge in the number and scale of events from about 1979/80 onwards, more and more new events focused on the half-marathon. The arithmetical half had a clear logic to it, and indeed many new marathon events used a two-lap course, whereby half-marathons ended after a single lap. Many of the traditional 10-mile races were in areas where traffic had increased substantially, with all the associated practical difficulties and extra costs. So the trend has been a gradual decline in 10-mile races and a growth in half-marathons. This has coincided with a shift towards professional event management companies taking on the events where participant numbers run into the thousands, although of course the 'traditional' club-based races organized by volunteers still exist across the country.

A particularly British trend has been that the sheer scale and public profile of the London Marathon has made it financially challenging for many second-tier marathons to stay afloat, as many thousands of people enter London and if not accepted they simply do not carry on training as there is no other marathon that they are drawn to. The likes of Holland, Spain, Italy and Germany have maybe a wider spread of quality marathons. However, the encouraging growth in the UK of new marathons such as Edinburgh and Brighton, backed up by proven stalwarts such as Belfast, Nottingham, Lochaber and Abingdon, offers a healthy range of options across the main marathon seasons of spring and autumn. At the time

of writing, Liverpool and Manchester are also resurrecting marathons that had been run in previous decades but had fallen by the wayside of other urban pressures.

Modern trends of globalization, budget airlines and, for most, increasing disposable income, lead to many people now taking a more international approach to their running plans, particularly for marathons. Chapter 11 suggests a few options beyond the global big hitters.

This isn't a travel guide but the international angle does have a few points relevant to running performance.

It means that the marathon and half-marathon season in Europe becomes longer. The biggest events invariably try to avoid the most extreme weather in their respective countries. So the trend is that in Northern

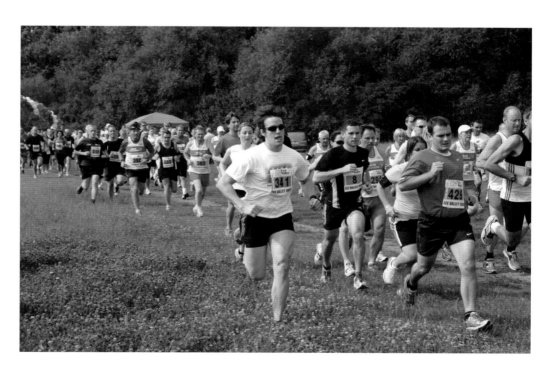

Many road races may use some off-road surface on the course.

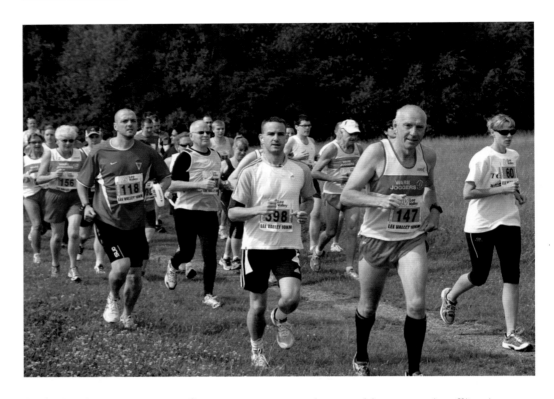

A typical road-racing cross-section of seniors, veterans, men and women, club runners and unaffiliated.

Europe and Scandinavia the main marathons are held around June, as any earlier would risk extreme cold weather for much of the training build-up of the domestic runners. Travel south to Italy and Spain and they tend to opt for February/March and then an autumn block in November, using dates when difficult hot weather is unlikely to be a factor. It is like a modern version of the eighteenth-century's Grand Tour, with a higher aerobic challenge but fewer highwaymen.

These extended seasons mean that for a race-greedy marathoner the options are increased. For example, one could go for Seville in early February, London in mid/late April, Helsinki in early August and Florence in late November. It's a demanding schedule and although not insane it's unlikely to be optimum for performance. However, such a schedule would allow for four structured cycles of preparation with a progression from recovery through transition, then event-specific training, then taper, race and start the recovery again. More on this in Chapter 4.

Other Long-Distance Races

It is also worth clarifying at this stage that for the purposes of this book, we are looking at marathons and half-marathons as standard road events held entirely or almost entirely

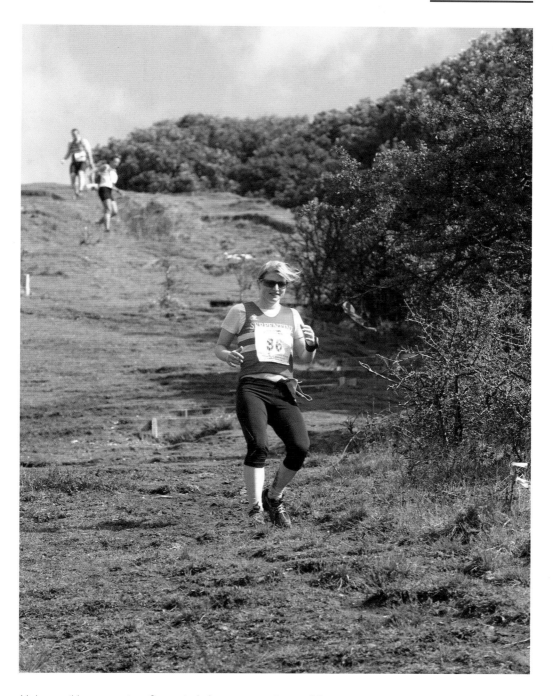

Make sensible preparations for particularly extreme racing conditions.

on a normal road surface. Also, although many events will be undulating to some degree, this book does not consider mountain races or even long-distance hill races. These are addressed in excellent and expert detail in Sarah Rowell's Crowood book *Off-Road Running*.

Of course, there is considerable common ground in training for and competing in what are all long-distance running races, but also enough specific differences to treat them as separate disciplines. As an example, when the leaders of a 20-minute hill race can split their race into 16 minutes for the climb and 4 minutes for the descent, there are clearly factors somewhat different from that even-ness of effort that 'normal' road races are built upon. Indeed, within the National Governing Body structure there are distinct associations for fell and mountain running.

For runners who are in a phase of general training — as described in Chapter 4 — it can certainly be both physically beneficial and mentally invigorating to try some of these 'off the beaten track' events. But if you choose to do so, put some thought into including some pre-event training sessions to prepare your body for the unaccustomed severity of the uphill and downhill sections. Quads, calves and glutes will all take a battering, so take steps to ensure that they are not so trau-matized post-race that a return to training is unduly delayed.

With marathons and half-marathons at the top end of the standard endurance-running event group, you should definitely look more holistically at a varied and structured racing programme to include 10km, 5km races such as park runs, 10 miles and — if it is not too much of a culture shock tainted by ghastly school memories — cross-country in autumn and winter.

Another option that seems to be becoming ever more popular is the split loyalty between triathlons and long-distance running. From a purist perspective, a coach would invariably see running as the preferred aerobic training option to improve running performance. But coaches are obliged to work in the real world rather than a marathoning idyll. It is perhaps a subtle distinction, but the preference is to use triathlon as a valuable part of the general background for running, rather than vice versa. It is not an exact formula, but if you can find a three- to four-month block before a running target during which you focus on your running, that should strike a reasonable balance. Keeping a weekly swim and/or bike session going, at moderate intensity, during this phase, should also be enough to keep some tri-competence without impacting on your capacity for the running.

A further sign of the running times is the development of ultra running — 'ultra' being anything longer than the marathon distance, with 50km being the typical baseline for this category. The focus distances and events of the ultra world are 100km/62 miles and 24 hours, but there are almost endless options and variations of distances, surfaces, dura-tion and indeed location. Also bear in mind that although not officially classed as ultras, hilly off-road runs in the 20- to 25-mile range that take longer to complete than a standard marathon event are physiologically in the ultra ballpark.

As a general summary, the author suggests the following:

- If you are keen to see what you can achieve at marathon and half-marathon, ideally the ultra events are distances that you should tackle once you think you have achieved most of what you are capable of at the standard road distances. Even if you become involved in ultras whilst improving at marathon and half-mara-thon, you would probably improve more if you spared yourself the ultras. If you study the training recommendations and programmes used for ultra running, you will see why they are not really optimum for improving your speed over shorter endurance events, as there is so much emphasis on easing down for the long run, doing the long run, and recovering from the long run.

- If you wish to try your first ultra, block out a four-month window for the specific training; allow about four weeks to recover gradually from the event and get back into some easy regular running, then refocus on shorter events.

- The mental side of ultras becomes in many ways a different game from that which is applicable further down the endurance distances. Simplifying, for many it becomes about continuing to cover the distance at whatever pace, with actually finishing the event in itself a victory, whereas in this book we are looking at runners for whom completing a marathon or half-marathon is a given and the quality of the performance is the focus.

Whilst ultras are indeed a growth area of the sport, they remain a minority area, as the statistics for the number of people who tackle events beyond the marathon would confirm. The author ran some twenty marathons, was seen within the middle ranks of club distance running as a marathon specialist, yet never once wished to find out what a longer distance would be like. For further detailed insights into ultra running and training plans, the website www.halhigdon.com is informative and well respected.

Clubs and Training Groups

If this book had appeared twenty-five years ago, this subject matter would have been easy to cover. There were two options. Either you joined a traditional athletic 'Harriers' club, or you joined a 'new breed' runners club.

The Harriers club would be populated mainly by athletes with some level of natural talent, nearly all of whom would have been in the sport since secondary school. Most of them would train either daily or twice daily, with thorough but often quite informal links to experienced coaches, who had themselves come through a similar system. Those athletes who tackled marathons and half-marathons did so with a high degree of commitment, invariably having progressed through the endurance events starting at 800/1,500m, through 5km and 10km and then upwards. They nearly all did cross-country races as part of their running regime. These runners and coaches were mostly male; females, although starting to make their presence more widely felt from the early 1970s, were principally involved as cake bakers, sandwich slicers and kit washers. As context, in 1976 the longest Olympic running race for women was 3,000m, an inequality that went right down through the sport.

The new breed of running clubs had a huge growth spurt between 1980 and 1982, stimulated by initially the London Marathon, which arrived in April 1981, and then the massive spread of other long-distance road events described above. Members of these clubs were typically latecomers to the sport; often had little endurance prowess or more general athletic traits; had little interest in testing themselves across athletic events; and in the main did not have access to the sort of coaching wisdom held in the traditional clubs. In marked contrast to the Harriers, it was not uncommon to make their competitive debut over the full marathon distance, usually lacking the years of training that the average Harrier would take to their debut marathon.

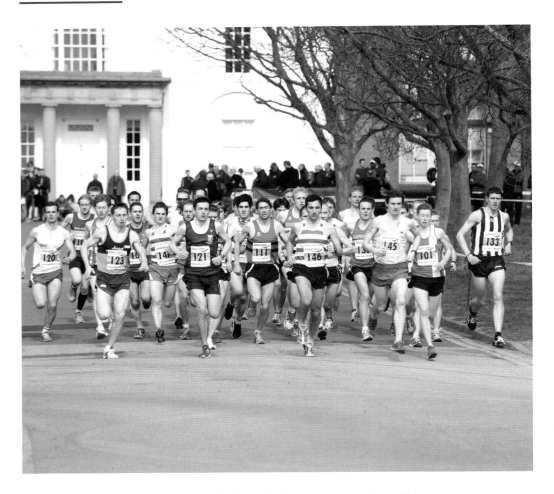

ABOVE AND OPPOSITE: When choosing a club, find one that best suits your running ambitions.

With the women's marathon joining the Olympics in 1984 after being included in the very first World Athletics Championships in 1983, the concept of women running long distances quickly played catch-up and membership of the new breed of clubs was more equally split between the genders.

Gradually, however, the distinctions between the two types of clubs merged. There was arguably an element of complacency and a lack of any succession planning at the peak of the British endurance scene in the mid-1980s – an assumption that we would always have swathes of lean, talented, ambitious young runners coming through, backed up by an even greater number of second-tier county-level runners. But through a combination of societal and political factors, the endurance-running world changed immensely and many clubs found fifteen years later that their squad of talented twenty-somethings had become a bunch of seasoned forty-somethings, with almost nobody following in their wake.

Meanwhile, within what the Harriers had previously perceived as 'jogging clubs', nuggets of athletics performance and coaching expertise had emerged. The new breeders learned that cross country was a great way to set the base for spring half-marathon and marathon races; that structured and periodized interval training, hard work as it was, could boost performance on top of what could be achieved just by long steady club runs from the pub car park; and that with a larger proportion of women in their member-ship, set against the relatively weaker standards in-depth in women's running, they could start to compete at national level against the traditional big hitters. The author recalls a road race in the mid-1980s where a Burnham Jogger ran 64.45 for a half-marathon, which certainly pushes the definition of jogging to a rather swift limit. Indeed, this performance is right in line with the qualifying time that many Federations use when selecting athletes to run in the World Half-Marathon Championships.

The developments of organized running within the current millennium include the likes of regular groups led by personal trainers operating out of gyms and fitness centres;

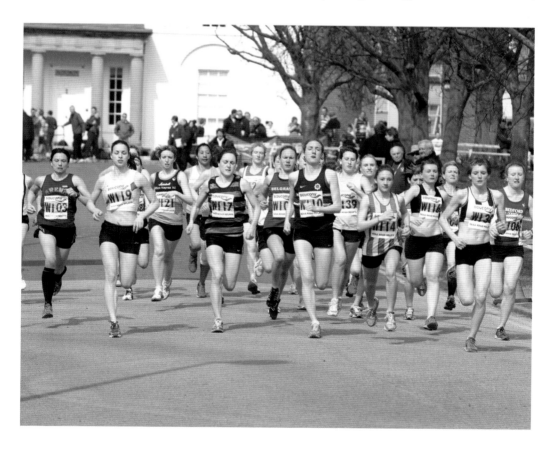

Run England groups led by qualified run leaders as an affiliated part of England Athletics, the National Governing Body for the sport; jogscotland programmes led under the auspices of the scottishathletics federation; corporate running groups where most of the training is done by colleagues during their time at the office; and 'virtual' groups or clubs where a coach or trainer develops a group ethos mainly by a website presence and maybe some actual group training days or warm weather training trips.

To the outsider, even the most modest running clubs might come across as being too 'elitist'. But as a general observation for people who may be worried about taking the step of joining a club, most running clubs will have more mid-pack or slower runners than you might guess. In general, the likelihood would be that having some sort of 'other people' structure around your running will make your time in the sport more enjoyable than if you did the whole thing in splendid isolation. And part of this benefit will be that you will probably end up with improved performances. You might also end up with a larger bar bill.

Do be choosy in joining a club or group where you find a good match with your own level of commitment and if this evolves over time, review the set-up. You will only ever be a twenty-seven-year-old newcomer, a thirty-five-year-old keen club runner, or a forty-seven-year-old dogged veteran once, so try to be in the optimum running environment. Avoid the scenario whereby you look back wistfully and wish you had linked up with Club X or Coach Y five years earlier.

KEY POINTS

- Do not underestimate what you can achieve if you are committed, consistent and train hard and smart.
- Be sensible about how you focus on triathlons, ultras, mountain or fell races if you are keen to make optimal progress in marathons and half-marathons.
- Consider the benefits of doing at least some of your training with a club or structured group.
- Do read the underpinning technical chapters in Part II to gain most from the training Chapters in Part I.

TRAINING AND RACING

CHAPTER 2

BASIC TRAINING PRINCIPLES

In this section, which many seasoned runners will be at least partly familiar with, we look briefly at how endurance running is fuelled; the key systemic changes we need to improve so as to aid long-distance performance; and introduce the overarching training structures to achieve these improvements. This sets the context for the more detailed training advice and schedules in subsequent chapters.

How It Works

In brief, the main energy form used in human muscle is adenosine triphosphate (ATP), a high-energy compound whose breakdown converts its chemical energy into mechanical energy, or muscle contraction. ATP is essential for the muscle to contract, but muscle stores of ATP are very limited, enough for a second or two at the most. For the muscle to continue to contract, ATP must be replenished. The speed at which you can continue to run depends on your ability to replenish ATP in your active muscles.

Sports scientists have classified three distinct human muscle energy pathways ranked in order of their ability to replenish ATP:

1. The adenosine triphosphate–phosphocreatine (ATP–PCr) energy pathway is designed to replace ATP very rapidly. Phosphocreatine (PCr) releases energy to synthesize ATP very rapidly, but, like ATP, PCr content in the muscle is also limited. The ATP–PCr energy pathway is predominant in very short duration, high-power events and lasts about eight seconds. It is therefore of almost negligible significance in fuelling long-distance running performance .

2. The lactic acid energy pathway, more technically known as anaerobic glycolysis, involves the rapid breakdown of muscle glycogen (glycolysis) under conditions when oxygen supply is limited (anaerobic). It replenishes ATP less rapidly but in greater quantities than the ATP–PCr energy pathway and is the predominant energy pathway in more prolonged sprints, such as 400m. Accumulation of lactate

(lactic acid) in the blood induces muscle fatigue, so the endurance of this energy pathway is somewhat limited. However, lactate itself is a powerful energy source and the painful effect caused by its accumulation is because it is stored with an attached hydrogen ion. This ion is acidic; it changes the pH level of the blood from its more alkaline nature and restricts the pathway of oxygen, thus leading to a rapidly increasing level of fatigue. Broadly, you can run in a predominantly anaerobic state for about 60–70 seconds, so that is obviously crucial in 800m and 1,500m races, but it becomes an ever decreasing part of performance as the race distance increases.

3. The oxygen energy pathway involves the aerobic metabolism of either carbohydrate (aerobic glycolysis) or fat (aerobic lipolysis), producing substantial quantities of ATP but at a slower rate than the other two pathways. The oxygen energy pathway predominates in longer aero-bic endurance events. Although both carbohydrate and fat may be used as fuel sources for the oxygen energy pathway, carbohydrate is the more efficient fuel. Carbohydrate produces more ATP per unit of oxygen than does fat.

Long-distance running depends primarily on the oxygen energy pathway. Its optimal functioning during long-distance events is dependent upon various body systems. For example, the digestive system is essential to provide fuel for muscular energy before and during performance. The endocrine system secretes hormones such as insulin and epinephrine that influence fuel supply to the muscle. The integumentary system, which includes the skin, is involved in temperature regulation, particularly important under warm environmental conditions.

However, the two key system combinations involved in the aerobic pathway are the neuromuscular and cardiovascular–respiratory systems. The neuromuscular system

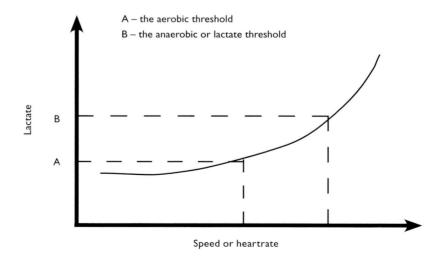

A – the aerobic threshold

B – the anaerobic or lactate threshold

The Lactate Curve.

(nervous and muscle systems), which consists of the brain, peripheral nerves and muscles, generates the muscular energy to run with the appropriate speed and efficiency. The cardiovascular and respiratory systems, which consist of the heart, blood vessels and lungs, provide oxygen, the keystone to the aerobic pathway.

The interaction of the neuromuscular and cardiovascular–respiratory energy systems determines several of the key components of running potential:

- **Maximal oxygen uptake (VO_2 max)** This measures the ability of the cardiovascular system to deliver, and the neuromuscular system to utilize, oxygen during running. It is related to bodyweight, so is expressed per kilogram of bodyweight.
- **The lactate threshold** (often referred to as the anaerobic threshold, perhaps less precisely because even at lower levels of effort there is an element of anaerobic energy being produced) This represents the level of running intensity at which energy production becomes increasingly anaerobic, leading to lactate accumulation in the blood and increased fatigue.
- **Running economy** This refers to the ability of the neuromuscular and cardiovascular–respiratory systems to maximize oxygen efficiency, obtaining the highest running speed for the amount of oxygen used. Speed represents the ability of the neuromuscular system to maximize energy production for running.

In general, improvement in any of these components will enhance endurance-running performance. Marathons and half-marathons are run at a pace just below the lactate threshold, so improving running economy, which is an increase in speed at a given oxygen uptake, is a key element.

What We Want From It

So you need to maximize, or at least improve, your ability in the above three parameters to progress your long-distance running performance. The training you do will:

- improve the cardiovascular system to transport blood and oxygen. Increases in heart pumping capacity, total blood volume and capillarization of muscle tissues are some principal changes induced through suitable training;
- improve the ability of the muscles to use oxygen effectively by converting carbohydrate and fat into ATP. Increases in the size and number of mitochondria, oxidative enzymes and myoglobin in oxidative muscle fibres are beneficial changes.

Collectively, these adaptations to training will:

- improve aerobic capacity (VO_2 max);
- improve the lactate threshold, so that it is attained at a faster running speed;
- improve running economy by lowering the energy demand of running; and
- improve speed, or the ability of the neuromuscular system to maximize energy production for running.

Mitochondria, developed by aerobic training.

How We Improve It

Before we look at how to build up the training specifics, it is helpful to ensure that we have a foundation in understanding the principles of why we train at all.

The usual rationale for the benefits of training is about adaptation and super-compensation. This applies to any sports training. Put simply, you challenge the body's limit of a particular performance factor, which then fatigues the body, giving it a short-term dip. It then gradually recovers, restores itself to the original level and then the 'super-compensation effect' adds a small margin of additional capacity at whatever element it has been challenged. It is also notable that different types of running session will have a beneficial effect on more than one parameter of endurance performance, as the table on page 35 shows.

Because regular training means training on most days, it is very hard to put a timeline on how long this process takes in full, because any hard training session will always have various other training stimuli on preceding and succeeding days, each with their own benefits. However, most experienced athletes and coaches think that it takes about ten to twelve days to get the full benefit of a training session. It follows therefore that when looking at a target race and planning a taper, particularly for marathons, you should go back about twelve days beforehand for your last key and race-specific training session. After this, the training focus should be on maintenance and avoiding detraining. If you look at how an elite athlete trained for a big race you should often see a big, hard, specific session about ten to twelve days out.

Rates of Improvement – The Genetic Lottery

It is also worth mentioning that a major factor in a runner's rate of improvement will be their individual make-up of slow-twitch and

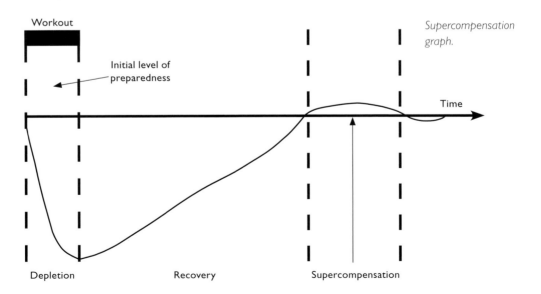

Supercompensation graph.

fast-twitch fibres. Simplifying for the sake of keeping the science relevant to what can be applied in practice, we have three types of muscle fibres:

- **Type 1** Slow twitch (red), best suited to aerobic energy production.
- **Type 2a** Fast-twitch oxidative (white), which can also be trained to take on the aerobic efficiency of Type 1 fibres, but if not trained aerobically are in essence used for more speed-based energy requirements.
- **Type 2b** Fast-twitch glycolytic, which use the anaerobic (glycolytic) energy system and cannot be adapted to operate aerobically.

The large majority of untrained people have a fast-twitch vs slow-switch balance that falls between 45 and 55 per cent of each type. The world elite are genetic outliers who have around 80 per cent slow twitch (long distance), or 80 per cent fast twitch (sprinters). The same trends would be apparent in other sports, depending on where the sport fits in the spectrum between speed and endurance.

It is not known exactly how the adaptation of Type 2a to Type 1 fibres occurs, nor is there any data that draws clear links between what a few extra per cent of slow-twitch fibres is 'worth' in performance terms. On a practical level, there is nothing you can do to change your composition of Type 2b fibres. What you may notice is that if you are training with others, a key factor in how quickly people improve their endurance performance, and indeed the level at which they level off when they are training at close to their maximum capacity, is how well-endowed they are with slow-twitch fibres.

Structured Improvement

This is where we now start crossing over from the scientist's domain into the coach's territory.

The flip side of the preceding point about training adaptations is that they are reversible. In simple terms, 'use it or lose it!' So, for example, if you do a hard session at your target half-marathon pace on Day 1 of a cycle, then sometime around Days 10 to 12 you will reap the benefit if you test yourself. But if you then neglect to challenge yourself again at that sort of intensity, the benefit from the effort made on Day 1 will start to seep away gradually. In the short term the amounts, if we expressed them either as a percentage or in seconds per mile or per kilometre, are small, and particularly so if we isolate them to just one training session, but over a few months the loss of event-specific fitness would become more striking.

There is no exact formula for the rate of performance decline, as there are so many variables on what can be done to give some sort of aerobic effort instead of structured training. The general trend is that in the short term – about five to ten days – the loss is very minimal. Then if there is a rest that extends into weeks and months the decline becomes much more marked.

On a practical planning basis one can see a link between the approximate time to absorb the benefit of a session and the fourteen-day training cycle around which many plans are structured. Broadly, this gives the athlete one session per cycle at each of the four or five main levels of intensity around which they are building their training.

Another cornerstone of training principles, and particularly for more seasoned runners, is that once the body has gone through a repeated cycle of a particular training stimulus, the response to that stimulus will, in the

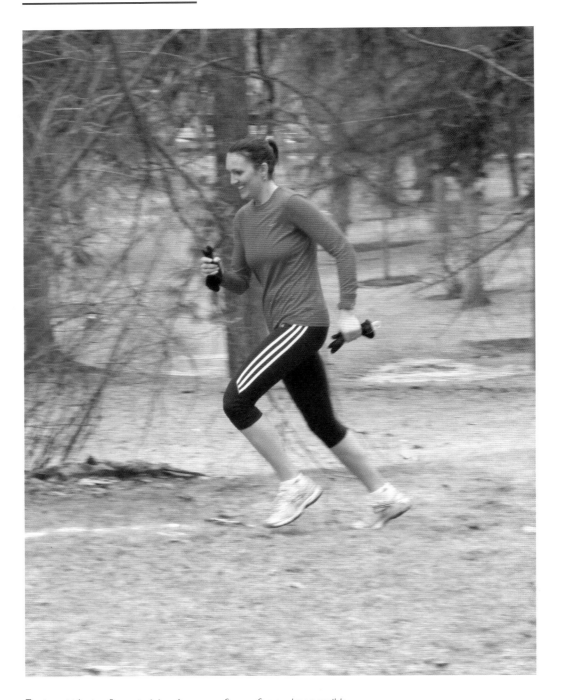

Try to get plenty of your training done on softer surfaces when possible.

short term, probably have been maximized. There is likely therefore to be greater benefit in doing something different and drawing the benefit from a new stimulus. We are considering this all within the context of what is of performance benefit to endurance running, so when talking of variety we do not mean sideline the threshold running and have a basketball practice instead.

A simple and relevant example could be that if you have spent eight weeks building up your long run from, say, 10 to 20 miles, all at similar steady pace, there should then follow a similar period where the focus is about doing comparable distances at greater speed. Of course, if you repeat the same long run of, say, 14 miles week in week out, there may still be considerable benefit and indeed you may do some pace variations within it on a 'how you feel on the day' basis, but the rate of progress is likely to be slower than if you are more systematic in following good practice.

The author's experience is that for many seasoned and committed runners who are sensibly 'ticking the boxes' of the main physiological factors in long-distance running (and it is somewhat unfair to consider someone who may run 70 miles per week as a mere aerobic box ticker), the single most useful coaching benefit to add to their programme is a purposeful use of periodization. Put simply, this involves seeking to optimize the balance of each training stimulus so that nothing is left undercooked, nor is anything pursued past the point at which it continues to add value. There most definitely is not a formula for this that works for all runners all of the time. Whoever finds that formula can be the proud author of what would be the last endurance coaching book ever needing to be written.

Six-Month Macrocycle – The Full Season

Mesocycle 1 – transition	Mesocycle 2 – general endurance 1	Mesocycle 3 – general endurance 2	Mesocycle 4 – specific endurance 1	Mesocycle 5 – specific endurance 2	Mesocycle 6 – peaking and competing

Each microcycle comprises a fourteen-day block of training and recovery

Microcycle 1 – recovery	Microcycle 3 – steady running/ threshold	Microcycle 5 – steady running/ threshold/ vVO$_2$ max/ hills	Microcycle 7 – steady running/ long distance/ marathon pace/ hills	Microcycle 9 – steady running/ long distance/ marathon pace/ 5km/10kmpace	Microcycle 11 – peaking for event steady running/ threshold/ marathon pace/vVO$_2$ max
Microcycle 2 – transition	Microcycle 4 – steady running/ threshold/vVO$_2$ max	Microcycle 6 – steady running/ threshold/vVO$_2$ max/hills	Microcycle 8 – steady running/ long distance/ marathon pace/ 5km/10km pace	Microcycle 10 – steady running/ threshold/ marathon pace/ 5km/10km pace	Microcycle 12 – taper/ competition

Within these cycles, periodic recovery and 'absorption' weeks should be planned.
NB: Whilst VO$_2$ max is the measurement of maximum oxygen intake, vVO$_2$ max is the actual running speed (v = velocity) that corresponds to this level of oxygen intake

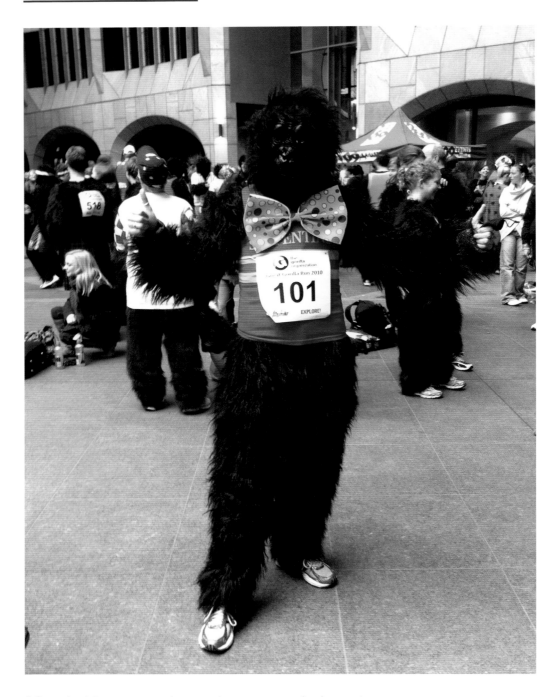

A focused training programme does not rule out some more low-key running events.

If we break down how a six-month season targeting a marathon might look, going from the headline to the progression of the fortnightly cycles, but not yet drilling down to a daily detail, we arrive at something like the structure below. A few key points to bear in mind:

- We will assume that Day 1 is the day after a target marathon or half-marathon and that the final day, Day 168, is the next target marathon.
- These cycles can apply whether one is running three, four, five or more times per week.
- There is no 'difficult' running until the fifth week and this is no quicker than about a 10-mile race pace.
- Useful and important as it most definitely is, there is no 'traditional' interval training until about the seventh week, at which point some relatively short bursts, in the region of 40–60 seconds, can be introduced.
- There is no structured or extended running at target race pace until about the fourth month, although in practice there is no harm in 'dabbling' with this in some parts of some long runs.
- 'Long distance' means further than about 16 miles, which is viewed by many as the 'cut-off point' beyond which only marathon specialists gain additional training benefit.
- There is no harm in mixing different stimuli within one session as long as you know what you are doing and why, so a set of short hill reps can be sandwiched between some stints at threshold, or a bout of half-marathon pace alternated with shorter stints at 10km race pace.

Most runners will find that once every three or four weeks they will benefit from reducing the training load by about one-third from the previous month's peak. This will apply to both volume and intensity. So, for example, if your weekly mileage has been 40 on average, just under 30 should be planned. You should similarly cap the harder training sessions, whatever their composition, at about two-thirds of what would be a full, challenging session. This usually gives the right balance between maintaining fitness, whilst avoiding the risk of overtraining and preventing any detraining. This downsizing should also be reflected in your strength and conditioning session(s) in the relevant week.

Of course, any number of factors such as work, domestics, even shifting around the days on which you do your long run, may prevent this reduced week being an exact arithmetical two-thirds. Do not agonize over the numbers, but do try and get an overall feel that the week feels like a noticeable 'freshen-up' phase. It is fairly common and logical practice to try to match these easier weeks to those that end with a race you wish to do well in.

At this point it is worth noting that amidst all the training intensities and session options, there is no magic-wand effect that interval training produces for experienced or improving runners. Whilst it is no doubt true that if all your running is at what you find either a slow or a steady comfortable pace, then interval training – running faster repetitions at something close to 100 per cent of your VO_2 max with a managed recovery between each fast effort – will definitely bring performance improvements more quickly and more substantially than doing the same steady state stuff day in day out. All distance runners should make use of this training, although not all will enjoy it.

But beware of thinking you need to do these sessions week in, week out, all year round. If we are talking about 'classic' interval sessions, where the fast stretches are between, as a minimum, about 40 seconds and extending to about 4 minutes maximum (beyond which the pace would drop slightly for a slightly different training purpose), then in a six-month macrocycle as outlined above, there may be between about eight and ten such sessions so it need not be a weekly penance. And for long-distance races you should definitely not need to do more than one such session in a week.

As one UK national coach said of the British long-distance elite from the 1970s and 1980s: 'Looking at the training diaries, before Christmas it was just a set of numbers of miles, not much of a training structure.' No criticism was implied, or taken; the point being made was that in order to make the most of a more selective and periodized series of interval sessions, the underlying aerobic base should be prioritized.

Coaching Support

By reading this book you are clearly taking an additional step in your coaching set-up. At the two extremes of coaching we would see at the very simplest level a totally self-contained, poorly informed runner who does all his training 'by feel' with no knowledge of the relevant training practices. At the most complex and precise we would find the Olympic champion, who would have a professional coach, probably funded by the National Governing Body, to pay close attention to him on a daily basis. The coaching set-up would be backed up by sports doctors, scientists, a nutritionist and a psychologist, and each time the athlete took part in a major event someone would have recced the event details on an athlete's behalf. The sort of detail checked out on British athletes' behalf at the Olympic Games

includes the distance from the warm-up track to the final call room and the electricity current in the hotel rooms.

Only a tiny number of athletes operate in this rarified world of full-time elitism. Similarly, it is increasingly hard to imagine in the developed world a runner wishing to improve without some sort of research using the Internet, books, magazines, or of course the old-fashioned option of actually speaking to people with some knowledge and experience. A good coach should nearly always be able to add something to an athlete's performance. The level of input and the measurement of the benefit will vary in every individual case.

If you think about the value of coaching support in the long term then maybe its merits become more demonstrable. Let's suggest that a good coach can be worth an average of 1 per cent per year to an athlete's results. Typically, the benefit would be greater at the outset and would reduce as the athlete becomes more experienced, knowledgeable and starts to get closer to their physical limit. This hypothetical 1 per cent is the 'added value' that comes on top of what the athlete may be doing based on their own ideas regarding issues such as increasing mileage, structured sessions and strength and conditioning. If you do the maths on a four-year cycle, that 4 per cent at 7 minutes per mile, at race pace, gives about 17 seconds per mile, so about 3 minutes in a half-marathon and 7 minutes in a full marathon. Maybe food for thought if you are a self-coached 3.07 marathoner who has reached a plateau.

If you have a PhD in exercise physiology, have read widely, have a reflective nature and are in a high-performance athletics club, the coaching margins may be smaller. But if you are relatively new to the sport, have not yet found a suitably holistic and individualized package of coaching wisdom on websites or in magazines, and are doing all your planning isolated from a running club structure, then coaching benefits may be greater for you.

In addition to the more obvious staples of a training plan and technical knowledge, there are more subtle benefits that a coach may bring. These include:

- Motivation. Not in the obvious sense of an in-your-face Mr/Ms Motivator, but the runner's awareness that the coach has spent a fair amount of time putting together a training plan, so you should feel a level of obligation to follow it if you are fit and able to do so.
- Quality-assured recommendations to, for example, masseurs, physiotherapists or osteopaths and podiatrists. Sometimes it seems that everybody in the medical services sector claims extensive expertise on 'sports injuries', but the number with good credentials on the specifics of endurance running is somewhat smaller and a coach can help steer you in the right direction.
- Links to training partners or groups, particularly for long runs and harder sessions, where the presence of others is invariably worth a few seconds per mile compared to doing it all solo, when your mind has nothing to focus on apart from the increasing fatigue.
- Also, simply a 'third eye'. We've all had the experience of writing something like a CV or report where we've double, triple and quadruple checked it for accuracy and are convinced it is spot on, and then when a fresh pair of eyes reads it they pick up some typos or spelling errors. Sometimes we tell ourselves what we want to be told and our mind plays little tricks on us. A similar scenario can occur in running training, where a runner draws up a plan but has a blind spot.

Another coaching benefit can be to draw in the reins on the ambitious over-reacher. A typical scenario would be a runner who has made good progress and is starting to run a challenging volume of mileage, say 60 miles weekly in seven runs. It is very easy to sit down and write an ambitious plan to add, maybe, one-third across the board and push it up to 80 miles per week. The likelihood is that in the short term this sort of leap would be unsustainable and some combination of injury, illness or underperformance would occur. In general, with ambitious runners the coach may often err slightly on the side of caution and would not endorse a training regime that they suspected would increase the injury risk. Runners are perfectly capable of picking up injuries without a coach's input.

The flip side of the motivational angle can be that the coach should help you to keep the running in perspective if you have a tendency to become too fixated on its importance. If you have targeted say, sub-85 minutes for a half-marathon and you cross the line in 86.30, then it's a safe bet that your family, employment and social life will stay exactly as they were before the race. So whilst it will be useful to have an objective methodical reflection on what may not have gone right on the day, keep this disappointment separate from everything else in life and once you have found some learning points from the disappointment, move on.

If you are able to gain the advice of a coach, keep in mind the following guidelines:

- Give the coach at least three months and ideally six months to 'make a difference' unless you have a major and profound disagreement with the approach early on. Any competent coach wishing to reduce your risk of injury will evolve your training gradually, however enthusiastic you may be to revolutionize your approach overnight, and there is also a time lag needed to do the training, adapt to the benefits and perform faster.

- Seek a suitable match between your level of commitment and ambition and the coach's, otherwise one or both of you may soon become frustrated.
- Agree with the coach the frequency of communication that is likely to work best and what level of detail is needed to inform the progression of your training. The minutiae of whether you had a third piece of toast for breakfast, or whether your threshold run lost 57 seconds because of red traffic lights, can probably be kept to yourself, but a weekly or fort- nightly update is usually helpful for both parties.
- In an increasingly contract-based society, voluntary sports coaching has very few mutual obligations as long as the coach acts within what the relevant coach- ing licence's code of conduct requires. The world of sports coaching is certainly changing its shift between voluntary and paid coaches. There are no absolute rights and wrongs regarding what model works best, but the principles of good coaching, across the technical, communication and behavioural aspects, should be followed as well as possible whether the coach is working for a fee or as a volunteer.

KEY POINTS

- Remember that running economy complements and underpins training to improve your VO_2 max and lactate threshold.
- Aerobic and cardiovascular training bene- fits are reversible.
- Build in periodic maintenance weeks of training, however enthusiastic you are and however well you are progressing.
- A periodized training and racing plan should help your sense of purpose and motivation in addition to its physiological benefits.
- Evolution rather than revolution is the most effective way to progress your training.

CHAPTER 3

TRAINING – GENERAL ENDURANCE PHASE

'The road to anything worthwhile isn't going to be easy, and it shouldn't be.'

John Wooden,
Legendary USA basketball coach

Physiological Basics of the Events

We shall start with a reminder of the energy requirements of the various endurance events. Some readers may be surprised to learn that the Governing Body of the sport (International Association of Athletics Federations – IAAF) officially treats 'endurance running' as all events from 800m upwards, and National Governing Bodies follow suit. This impacts upon national and regional club structures, coaching, competitions and, filtering down to an individual level, it means a significant amount of common ground shared by 800m runners and mara-thoners, even though the latter is some fifty-two times the race distance. The main common feature, which the table below illustrates, is that the main energy source is aerobic and this is why the endurance event group is defined as it is.

It should be noted that these figures will vary slightly depending on what test proto-col is used and also that those shown below are based on high-performance runners. The slower the runner is over a given race distance, the higher the aerobic percentage will become, because with the anaerobic element only able to be sustained for a very

Energy Requirements for Different Endurance Events

Event	Aerobic Energy %	Anaerobic Energy %	ATP %
800m	40	51	9
1,500m	67	28	5
3,000m	82	16	2
5,000m	90	9	1
10,000m	95	4	<1
Half-marathon	98	2	<1
Marathon	99+	<1	<1

short time, the longer the race duration, the less proportion can be spent in an anaerobic state. So the aerobic/anaerobic energy split of a 50-minute 10km runner will be more in line with an elite half-marathoner than an elite 10km runner. Perhaps the main training element where mid-pack long-distance runners go astray from the event's requirements is either in doing too much anaerobic training or in putting too much store in how they may perform in the occasional anaerobic training that they do. Remember, your lactate tolerance at above your anaerobic threshold level will only show in the final 60–90 seconds of performance, therefore the further up the race distances you go, the less significance it will have. So, showboating at the end of a 400m interval session will not help you to sustain target pace in mile 11 of a half-marathon.

Which Training Paces for Which Benefits?

The table below shows the relative benefits of respective training paces, going from the easiest recovery pace to the most full-on speed work, and giving a relative weighting for each pace against each criterion you are trying to improve. The overall message to take away should be that even when you have a particular focus for a particular run, you will be ticking more than one performance box. There is clearly a mixture of art and science in putting together the optimum combination of these factors – and it is the 'art' bit that means you will not find any perfect set of numbers that will tell you exactly how to structure every part of every training run or session.

Another factor to bear in mind is that these physiological zones are often presented in an elite athlete context, so, for example, velocity at VO_2 max (or vVO_2 max) is often simplisti-

cally described as '3km race pace'. That's fine if you are Mo Farah, clicking off seven laps of the track at 60 seconds each, but for many runners their vVO_2 max will be far closer to their 1 mile/1,500 race pace. Even for a 38–40 minutes 10km runner it will correspond more closely to their notional 2km race pace. And so it is with the sort of physiological parameters allocated to elite runners' 10km and marathon race paces.

The training schedules in these chapters are seen as the best balance of mixing these factors for a certain level of runner aiming at the half-marathon and full marathon distances.

Planning

This is s a fundamental but often overlooked, or at the least, undervalued element of training for improved performance. For anyone who goes on an endurance coaching course it is a prominent feature throughout and it covers everything from planning a single run or training session to a long-term career plan. Of course, much of the skill is transferrable from sports training to any other aspect of life and so the content is often not entirely new to people.

Cliché as it is, 'fail to plan, plan to fail' is nevertheless very relevant. To put this in a long-distance running context, reflect on the earlier comments about periodization and consider the following. At a UK Athletics Marathon squad weekend for the nation's leading runners and coaches, the then Head of Endurance said 'If you don't draw up a plan that works back from your target race then I don't see how you can be confident that you will cover all the training that you need to cover to be thoroughly prepared.' (This man has coached Olympic medallists and was Mo Farah's long-term coach before Farah moved to the USA, so is as good as we will find.) It

Benefits of Different Training Paces

	Recovery/ Easy	Steady/ Comfortable slightly slower than Marathon Pace	Steady/Less Comfortable – quicker than Marathon Pace	10-mile to Half-Marathon Pace	10km to to 10-mile Pace	vVO$_2$ max – 2–3km Race Pace	Faster than 1,500m Race Pace
Increased blood volume	*	****	****	***	*		
Stimulates aerobic enzymes		***	***	***	****	*	
Stimulates fatty acids as fuel source	*	****	***	**	*		
Improved use of lactate as a fuel				**	***	***	****
Increased maximum rate of muscle glycogen usage				**	****	****	***
Increased capillarization	*	***	****	***	***	**	*
Improved blood and muscle buffering capacity				**	***	****	****
Increased maximum cardiac output			*	**	***	***	****
Increased ventilatory capacity				*	***	****	****
Improved neuromuscular adaption		*	*	***	****	***	***

**** maximum effect   *** very strong effect   ** significant effect   * limited effect is a telling point and one that many runners fail to address, in that it is too easy to start from the Now, Day Zero, and work forwards. Of course, simply starting with the end date and working backwards does not guarantee anything, but if you combine this with a thorough knowledge of the training principles and sessions, it is a big step towards putting together something coherent on Day Zero to get you to the key race date, which may be Day 154.

Admittedly, it can be somewhat daunting to draw up the full preparation macrocycle, say twenty-two weeks of seven days per week, and then to be faced with 154 blank spaces. But if you approach it systematically, things will fall into place. The order may take the following sequence:

- Insert the target race date(s).
- Add the other milestone races you plan to take part in, or at least the dates you plan to race if you have not yet entered specific events.
- At the top of the table split the twenty-two weeks into the phases of general training (say, eight weeks), event-specific training (twelve weeks) and taper (two weeks), as this will shape the further detail and assist you in planning the right sessions at the best stage.
- Insert any known days when running will not be possible because of whatever else may be going on in your life.
- Insert your most usual rest days. These may vary as life unfolds, but technically it is easy to put an R for 'rest' into a table. Indeed, if you are a five days a week runner this in itself will take care of about 30 per cent of your plan.
- Typically, you will do your long runs at the weekend – or perhaps on a fixed day most weeks if you have weekend commitments that prevent this. Insert the long run day

accordingly, before you add the detail of how these runs evolve.

- Logically and indeed based on the science of recovery from harder training efforts, the day after your long run will be a recovery day and in most cases so will the day before it, so add these. Again, the detail can follow; it could vary individually from 'nothing' to '2 × 5 mile easy runs'.
- Add in the usual day(s) on which you do some strength and conditioning training. This will invariably be on a day without a hard running session or long run.
- On the basis that you will rarely, if ever, do hard running sessions on two consecutive days, you should now start having a well-formed framework combining races, long runs, recovery days and harder days.

That, in many ways, is the technically easy bit and the detail is where the more specific knowledge and experience comes in. But a couple of examples illustrate what we are looking for. In a twenty-two-week marathon cycle building up to a big city event, we would not place a 23-mile training run in Week 2 because physically we are unlikely to be ready for such effort at this stage – at least, at a pace that is of training benefit. Nor (please!) would we do the run at the end of Week 21, because we would understand that so close to the marathon race it would leave the runner weary and under-recovered on marathon day.

Or consider a hard hill session, say twenty reps of 30 seconds up a challenging grass or off-road hill. We would be unlikely to tackle such a session at the beginning of Week 1 because we would not have had the build-up to make such a session manageable. Nor would we be best served by doing such a session at the end of Week 20 – two weeks before tackling 26 miles of flat tarmac we should not be focused on a session where

Cross-country running can be an effective but challenging way of building up endurance.

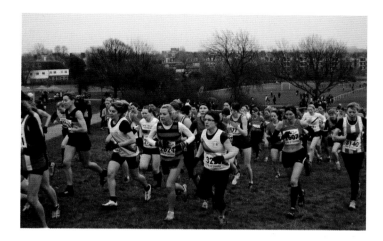

the fatigue is caused by a stimulus so remote from what we will be facing in the marathon.

And so on, with the details of the runs and sessions, until you arrive at something like the schedules shown later in this book.

Amidst all of this planning rigour, let's not lose sight that running is your leisure activity, not your job, and the bottom line is that it must add to your quality of life, not drag it down. So there may occasionally be spells when the training and racing plan, albeit valid and well intentioned, may come to feel like a burden rather than a support. At such times, do reflect on your level of enthusiasm and if you genuinely feel that a phase of running 'as you feel' would help recharge the motivational batteries, then go for the unstructured option for as long as it takes. If there is a coach involved, make the coach aware of this.

Chances are that if you continue to run regularly, the sheer monotony of doing every run at even pace and the same distance will soon become mundane and you will probably start introducing some sort of more performance-based structure to your running, with the key – and liberating – difference being that there is no external or pre-imposed pressure to do any of it; you just head out the door

and make the training up as you go along. Of course, you would still need to incorporate sound training principle within your DIY schedule.

General Training Cycle

We can now look further at the period between when you are recovered from the previous target performance, whether a marathon or shorter endurance race, and the training period for the next marathon or half-marathon target. We will use a block of about twelve to thirteen weeks. There is nothing sacred about this timescale and indeed for those who have target races that are more than six or seven months apart, the general training phase should be extended accordingly.

However, few runners will have the long-term patience to wait for close on a year between target races. At the other extreme, if we reduce the period between peaks, we start eating into the time available to make real improvements. So six months is a typical balance and is consistent with the principles described in Chapter 2. Generalizing somewhat, it also broadly mirrors the

British and indeed European road-racing season, with the main clusters of races falling around March/April and then in September/October.

The benefits you are looking for in this general phase will include:

- Overall, building back into regular running and harder training after some planned downtime.
- Working on pushing out the VO_2 max, initially with manageable sessions before increasing the length of the repetitions.
- Training at or around your lactate threshold, again starting with a modest challenge and building the duration. (It is worth noting that although this underpins endurance performance across the spectrum of distances, for 10-mile races and slightly shorter or longer, it is actually the specific race pace.)
- Improving your strength/strength-endurance via a suitable conditioning schedule. Logically, if you wish to improve your longer distance race performances, then whatever level of strength-endurance makes you 'fit for purpose' needs to be raised accordingly. Whilst the actual endurance-running training is being built up during this phase, it follows that there is some extra capacity to focus on the conditioning.

Hill training, depending on the detail of the sessions, can help to progress all of the above elements. For hill reps focused on strength-endurance and running at close to your heart rate at VO_2 max, use a hill (or part of a hill) of between 4 and 8 per cent gradient and run hard up it for 25–30 seconds. Turn around and jog back – the recovery between each rep should be about 45 seconds. The longer gaps between the sets are to enable the speed and intensity to be kept up but without an unhelpful build-up of excess lactate – an easy jog between sets should help to dissipate the lactate. Follow the last rep with seven to ten minutes of easy running on flattish terrain. Preferably do this session on a surface other than pavement – even a treadmill is better than paving stones. With hills, as with any other sort of repetition running, the duration of the effort, the number of repeats, and the duration and nature of the recovery can all be varied according to the main purpose. Try to avoid repeating in a hill session a stimulus that is too similar to another session in the same week of training.

As one leading British coach said, 'During the general phase, we aren't 800m runners or marathoners, we are all just endurance runners.' There is real wisdom in this statement and it is perhaps best exemplified in the training principles of Arthur Lydiard, the legendary New Zealand coach of the 1960s, who in many ways kick-started the training structures of endurance running that are still followed. The detail has certainly evolved somewhat and very few of the world's best follow a 'pure' Lydiard system, but all experienced coaches will have their roots in his ideas.

Because you are at this stage not in a specific mode, your race choices as far as distance and frequency can be less precisely planned. But be reasonable about this. Do not throw in a random marathon or 20-mile race without being prepared to do yourself justice, and use common sense and variety so that you are not, for example, racing frequent 10kms with the intervening sessions all focused on 10km pace. If you look back at the aerobic and anaerobic splits of the events from 3–5km up to the marathon, you can see that the schedules below lend themselves well to developing the major aerobic capacity needed for all these events, particularly when you are still more than three months before the target race(s).

Level One Schedule

- Throughout these schedules, 'easy' means about 65–70 per cent of maximum heart rate/effort, a pace at which you could carry out a normal conversation.
- 'Steady' means mid to high 70 per cent of maximum heart rate/effort, a pace where you can still talk but with slightly less ease.
- Mileage totals – calculations include about 2.5 miles for combined warm-up and warm-down for the harder sessions.
- Pace guide for faster sessions – the rule of thumb is that if you double the race distance, you add about 20 seconds per mile for what is a sustainable pace. Whether you are using a garmin, heart-rate monitor, or a more intuitive perceived effort, do try to work to these guidelines. If you do the first part of a session significantly too fast, the rest of the session will be compromised and you will lose much of the intended benefit, as well as missing the opportunity to develop your pace judgement, which is so essential in longer races.

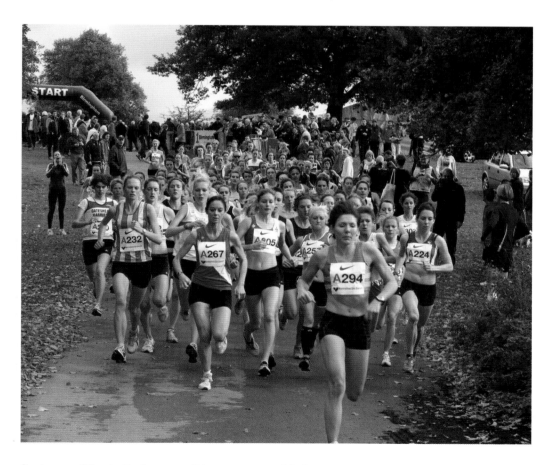

Short races of 5km to 5 miles are useful means to an end for longer races.

Level One Schedule

Day	Week 1	Week 2	Week 3	Week 4	Week 5	Week 6
1	40min easy inc 6 × 20sec strides	45min easy inc 6 × 20sec strides	45min easy inc 6 × 20sec strides	30min easy inc 6 × 20sec strides	35min easy inc 6 × 20sec strides	40min easy inc 6 × 20sec strides
2	45min steady	50min steady	w/up – 35min at threshold or slightly slower	w/up – 25min at threshold or slightly slower	w/up – 40min at threshold or slightly slower	w/up – long threshold reps – 5 × 7min with 75sec jog recovery
3						
4	45min steady	50min steady	w/up – 15min steady, then 20min alternating 30sec at notational 3km pace with 30sec jog recovery – w/down	w/up – fartlek on undulating course – 2 sets of (30sec–1–2–3 min) at 3km pace with 90sec recovery after each rep – w/down	w/up – fartlek on undulating course – 2 sets of (1–2–3–4min) at 3km pace with 90sec recovery after each rep – w/down	w/up – hill reps of 2 × 5 × 25sec climb, jog back recovery and 2min jog between sets
5						
6	Shorter of 9 miles or 80min	Shorter of 10 miles or 90min	Shorter of 12 miles or 1hr 45min	Shorter of 9 miles or 80min	Shorter of 12 miles or 1hr 45min	Shorter of 12 miles or 1hr 45min
7						
Total running miles	24	27	32	23	29	28

Day	Week 7	Week 8 (easier week)	Week 9	Week 10	Week 11	Week 12 (easier week)	Week 13
1	45min easy inc 6 × 20sec strides	30 min easy inc 6 × 20sec strides	40min easy	45min easy inc 6 × 20sec strides	45min easy inc 6 × 20sec strides	30min easy inc 6 × 20sec strides	45min easy inc 6 × 20sec strides
2	w/up – long threshold reps – 4 × 9min with 90sec jog recovery	w/up – long threshold reps – 5 × 8min with 80sec jog recovery	w/up –hill reps of 3 × 5 × 25sec climb, jog back recovery and 2min jog between sets	w/up – 3 × 5min reps at 10km pace (60sec jog) plug 6 × 2min reps at 5km pace (60sec jog) – w/down	w/up – 10min at threshold (90sec jog) 5 × 4 pace (2min jog) – w/down	w/up – 2 × 8min at threshold (90sec) + 3 × 5 min at 5km pace (2min jog) – w/down	w/up – 8 × 2min at 3km pace (75sec jog) + 35min at marathon pace (MP)
3							
4	w/up – hill reps of 2 × 6 × 25sec climb, jog back recovery and 2min jog between sets	30min easy	w/up – long threshold reps – 6 × 6min with 60sec jog recovery	w/up – hill reps of 2 × 8 × 25sec climb, jog back recovery and 3min jog between sets	w/up – hill reps of 3 × 6 × 25sec climb, jog back recovery and 2min jog between sets	40min easy	w/up hill reps of 2 × 9 × 25sec climb, jog back recovery and 3min jog between sets
5							
6	Shorter of 12/13 miles or 1hr 50min	10km race or XC race or time trial of 40min	Shorter of 13 miles or 1hr 50/55min	Shorter of 13 miles or 1 hr 50/55min	Shorter of 14 miles or 2hr	10km race or SC race or time trial of 40min	15 miles steady or 2hr 10min
7							
Total running miles							
	29	24	30	30	32	24	34

Level Two Schedule

Below is a slightly more advanced level of the same general principles. The key differences are as follows:

- There is a regular fifth weekly run, which accounts for about half the difference in the volume as compared to the plan above.
- The assumption is that the runner has just a bit more experience, capacity or commitment and so can slightly stretch out the weekly longer run; can handle slightly more voluminous and challenging hill sessions; and can sustain slightly greater volume at the quicker race paces.
- However, it is important not to unduly extend the amount of running that is

attempted at the paces that correspond to 3km/5km/10km pace, because beyond a certain volume or duration it just becomes physiologically impossible to keep the desired pace. The author recalls at a coach training course where someone suggested a session of four reps of five minutes at 1,500m race pace, which only becomes feasible if the recovery between repetitions becomes about one day.

Of course, there is nothing that stops runners from doing more than five runs a week in the general build-up, or exceeding 40 miles per week, which is the maximum that this plan builds up to. If you wish to head down a slightly more challenging path, the main changes to the plan would include:

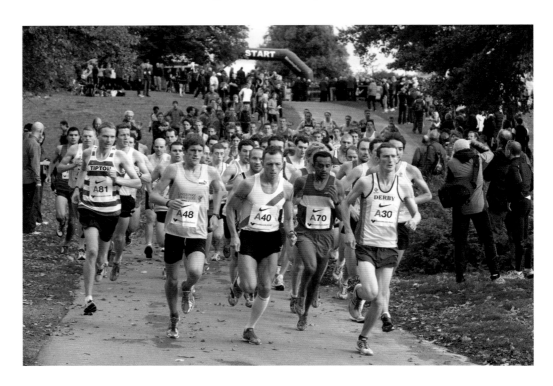

Some of these runners compete from 3k up to marathons.

- Add about 10–15 per cent to what is suggested to the long runs, so that before you start marathon specifics you have built up to some 16- or even 17-milers.
- Structure the longer runs to make them slightly more challenging than simply time on your feet, so that the latter few miles are approaching the sort of pace you would be targeting in the next marathon (or about 25 to 30 seconds per mile slower than half-marathon pace, if the marathon is not on your agenda).
- Add about 10–15 minutes to the 'bread and butter' steady runs, which will give a slightly greater boost to aerobic base building. But try to cap these steadies at 60 minutes; any longer and you are likely to start building up a muscular fatigue level that will adversely affect your capacity to do the following harder session at the planned pace.
- Add a sixth weekly run of about 40–45 minutes, as long as you are not losing the balance between quality and quantity by doing so.
- Consider adding a couple more races into the thirteen-week schedule. If you are doing all of the above in your regular training, you will be becoming pretty immersed in the sport and so more likely to wish to compete more regularly. Do vary the distances you tackle – if the baseline is 2 × 10km races, fill this out by adding a 5km race and either a 10-mile race or, if you have done the long runs to make the distance valid as a competitive effort, try a half-marathon towards the end of this phase.

If you include all of these additional training elements, you will typically be running about 50 miles per week, which – although in some ways this is just an arbitrary round number – is an approximate benchmark for serious club running. There are case histories in the following chapter showing how this can work.

Frequency of Marathons

We live in a running world where the marathon has for many people become much more than an athletic event. It can also fulfil people's ambitions on weight loss/management; international travel; charity fundraising; a lifestyle 'tick box' as in ' Twenty Things to Do Before You Are 40'; or indeed as part of preparation for a longer ultra running event or a triathlon Ironman. Amidst these different motivations one can lose sight of how best to make progress in one's marathon performance. On one hand, and particularly in London and south-east England, the London Marathon date can be the only one ever fixed upon by marathoners. Conversely, there are others who will get through maybe a dozen marathons a year, or in some cases more. We will stay focused on runners who wish to improve their marathon times and are looking for a marathon frequency to optimize their progress.

What is the best frequency? If you are in it for the long term, say at least five years, there is absolutely no harm in having a gap of a year or more between marathons if you continue to progress with your endurance training and racing in the meantime. You can make major aerobic advances in this spell and approach the next marathon from a much higher performance base. But if you wish to run more frequent marathons and to continue to improve consistently, let's look at what time frames are sensible.

In many ways, the overarching principles of recovery, transition, general training, specific training, taper and competition apply to a marathon as they do to an 800m runner, with a few specifics to reflect the sheer physical

Level Two Schedule

Day	Week 1	Week 2	Week 3	Week 4 (easier week)	Week 5	Week 6
1	50min easy inc 6 × 20sec strides	50min easy inc 6 × 20sec strides	55min easy inc 6 × 20sec strides	35min easy inc 6 × 20sec strides	45 min easy inc 6 × 20sec strides	40 min easy inc 6 × 20sec strides
2	50min steady	55min steady	w/up 35min at threshold or slightly slower	w/up – 25min at threshold or slightly slower	w/up – 40min at threshold or slightly slower	w/up – long threshold reps – 5 × 8min with 90sec jog recovery
3	40min steady	45min steady	40min easy		40min easy	40min easy
4	55min steady	60min steady	w/up – 15min steady – then 25min alternating 30sec at notional 3km pace with 30sec jog recovery – w/down	w/up – fartlek on undulating course – 2 sets of (30sec–1–2–3min) at 3km pace with equivalent recovery after each rep – w/down	w/up – fartlek on undulating course – reps of (1–2–3–4–5–4–3–2–1 min) at 3km pace for shorter reps. 5km pace for longer reps with 90sec recovery after each rep – w/down	w/up – 10min at threshold (2min jog) then hill reps of 2 × 6 × 25 sec climb, jog back recovery and 2min jog between sets
5				35min easy		
6						
7	11 miles steady	12 miles steady	13 miles steady	10 miles steady	13 miles steady	14 miles steady

Total running miles						
	35	39	39	29	38	38

Week 7	Week 8 (easier week)	Week 9	Week 10	Week 11	Week 12 (easier week)	Week 13
45min easy inc 6 × 20sec strides	30min easy inc 6 × 20sec strides	40min easy	45min easy inc 6 × 20sec strides	45min easy inc 6 × 20sec strides	30min easy inc 6 × 20sec strides	45min easy
w/up – long threshold reps – 4 × 10min with 2min jog recovery	w/up – long threshold reps – 5 × 7min with 90sec jog recovery	w/up – 10min at threshold then hill reps of 2 × 8 × 25 sec climb, jog back recovery and 2.5min jog between set	w/up – 3 × 6min reps at 10km pace (60sec jog) plus 7 × 2min reps at 5km pace (60sec jog) – w/down	w/up – 2 × 7min at threshold (60sec jog) 7 × 3min at 5km pace (90sec jog) w/down	w/up – 3 × 9min at threshold (90sec jog) then into 40min at target MP	w/up – 9 × 2min at 3k race pace (60sec jog) plus 40min at target MP
40min easy	30min easy			40min easy		45min easy
w/up 10min at threshold (2min jog) then hill reps of 2 × 7 × 25 sec climb, jog back recovery and 2.5min jog between sets	35min easy inc 1 × 3min effort at 10km pace	w/up – 2 × 10min at threshold (2min jog) then 4 × 4 min at 5km race pace with 2min jog recovery	w/up – 10min at threshold then hill reps of 3 × 6 × 25 sec climb, jog back recovery and 2min jog between sets	w/up – 10min threshold (2min jog) then hill reps of 2 × 9 × 25 sec climb, jog back recovery and 3min jog between sets	30min easy	w/up – 10min threshold (2min jog) then hill reps of 2 × 10 × 25 sec climb, jog back recovery and 3min jog between sets
		40min easy	45min easy			
14 miles steady	10km race or XC race or time trial of 40 min	14 miles progressive e.g. 3 miles easy – 7 miles steady marathon pace + 40–50 sec per mile – 4 miles at MP + 15sec per mile	15 miles steady	15 miles steady	10km race or XC race or time trial of 40 min	15 miles progressive e.g. 3 miles easy – 7 miles steady (marathon pace + 40–50 sec per mile – 5 miles at MP + 15secs per mile
39	28	38	39	39	29	42

challenge of a full-on marathon. Do bear in mind that, whilst the marathon is of course physically 'catabolic', in that in the short term it fatigues you immensely, in the bigger, longer-term picture it is an immense training effort. So, if you respect the recovery period, the marathon itself will be of use in shorter endurance races maybe four to six weeks later. If you can, try to avoid getting too immersed in your next marathon plan too soon after completing the last one, both physically and, just as importantly, mentally. It is hard to be a constantly committed marathon runner all year round. As a minimum, look at something like the following:

- **Week 1**   No running until at least five or six days after; maybe some very low-level, non-weight-bearing aerobic activity after about three or four days. Do not feel guilty about having a week off and limit any effort to about 40 minutes and about 70 per cent of maximum heart rate, that is, 'talking pace'. Massage about three to five days post-marathon may also be helpful in addressing some of the tightness that will have inevitably built up. Avoid massage in the 48 hours post-marathon, as your muscles will still be in a state of trauma.

- **Week 2**   Again, no harm in having a week off running and continuing to confine any 'training' to further low-level efforts of about 40 minutes of cross-training. Avoid the temptation of getting back into any regular group or club training at this stage. The recovery phase is gradual and does not recognize calendars or diaries, so after seven or fourteen days there will not be any major overnight rejuvenation. At the most, a 60- or 70-minute easy run on the weekend two weeks after the marathon can be attempted. Depending on your level of eating in this recovery phase, you may have gained a kilo or two of bodyweight for the obvious reason that your calorie requirements will have been somewhat less than when in training.

- **Week 3**   If you have been honest with yourself about allowing a real easy period in the previous fortnight, you may now feel ready to raise the training slightly. If so, then running on however many days per week was your marathon prep should be fine, but do spare yourself the rigours of intensity and long distance at this stage. As a guideline, about half of whatever has been your maximum weekly mileage should be manageable, with no need to run any of it quicker than your average marathon pace. This may be a suitable time to recommence some strength and conditioning.

So, three weeks later and if you have stayed at about racing weight, there should now be a balance between absorbing the major physical challenge of the marathon and the benefits it can bring to training, and allowing recovery and a level of regeneration from this immense effort.

As far as making further marathon progress, reflect on the duration of the training you did for the last marathon and think about what you will need to do to make some substantive difference to the performance level this achieved. If the marathon failed to go quite to plan in the later stages, and realistically this is often the case, do not see this as a lesser physical effort than the quicker time you had targeted. Any walking/slow jogging in the final miles was probably due to an overzealous pace in the preceding 15 or 20 miles, so even if you assess the result as disappointing, the physical impact still needs to be respected and absorbed.

It is notable that until the early 1980s the UK National Marathon Championships, which usually served as the main trial for any major international championships that summer (such as Olympic Games or European championships), were often held in late spring/early summer. The timeline from these domestic champs to the international event could be as little as nine or ten weeks and typically would be about twelve to sixteen weeks. As the science of marathon performance started to become more sophisticated during the late 1970s, leading coaches and athletes increasingly voiced their disapproval of what they considered inadequate recovery and regeneration time – and this may at least be partly linked to some British underperformances in the international races in this period. (We can't just simplify it as cause and effect though – there are too many variables in the marathon.) Also, it needs to be emphasized that even where results show that these top-level runners did successfully deal with two fast marathons maybe ten to twelve weeks apart, they would have had a good long-term planning structure in place to make this happen, and, importantly, this would be very much a one-off cycle and definitely not a recommendation to get into repeated marathon cycles of such short duration.

As far as some sort of minimum guidelines on what is needed to form the main body of the general and specific training, it is something like four weeks of general endurance work and four weeks of marathon specifics actually to make a difference. Bear in mind that a ten- to fourteen-day taper is needed to absorb the benefit of the harder training and convert it into marathon performance. Also, when looking at a relatively short gap between two marathons, remember that some of the specifics you did for the first marathon will – provided you have recovered sensibly – have a 'carry forward' effect for the second marathon. This would refer specifically to the very longest training runs. So, using a typical British marathon cycle as an example, if you have

done some very long runs through February and March for an April marathon, if you then do a July marathon, you should not need to replicate fully the menu of long runs through May and June.

So, putting these phases together, we are looking at about eleven or twelve weeks as a minimum time between two marathons, during which you can make discernible, but in all likelihood quite small, gains in your marathon potential. Of course, if the first marathon had gone much worse than expected, the second marathon may turn out significantly quicker, but this will probably be due to a much better pacing strategy rather than a massive short-term boost in actual underlying fitness.

If you do opt for a short cycle along the lines above, you would be well advised to have a longer gap before the next one, for example at least four months before you recommence specific marathon preparation.

Frequency of Half-Marathons

Clearly the extreme rigours of the final stages of the marathon are not – thankfully – shared by the half-marathon event. Many regular distance runners will do a long run of about 13 miles or more on almost a weekly basis. Physiologically, one could race a half-marathon every week of the year. The main restrictions might be the actual race calendar; how much time and money you wish to spend on transport costs and entry fees; and whether your wardrobe can withstand another fifty-two event T-shirts.

In terms of what will be best to improve your times, you should not stray too far from the principles of a planned macrocycle as described in Chapter 2. Broadly, you should follow these principles to make best progress – which is not to rule out that you may also improve in a non-target race if you are at a stage of developing your training and aerobic fitness anyway. Once you have chosen your target half-marathon, it may be helpful to put another benchmark half-marathon in your diary about eight or nine weeks earlier. For most runners, even well-conditioned marathon runners doing high mileage and regular long runs beyond 13 miles, they won't race a half-marathon that frequently, so it will be one of their longer races. As such, it is useful to get a robust indicator of half-marathon form en route to the target race. The eight- or nine-week window allows some decent time to recover and do a good block of further training to progress your fitness in a significant way.

Mental Aspects

The influence of the brain in running performance is seen by many within the coaching world as the biggest unexplored aspect. By and large, the physical and physiological aspects of endurance performance are believed to have been taken close to the limit in terms of what can be achieved. (Perhaps the most notable exception is 'gene doping', the genetic manipulation of individuals – which is not likely to be of practical relevance to this book's readership.) Of course, there may be some small gains to be made across various factors; randomly one could mention beetroot juice (see Chapter 9), alter G Treadmills (a very expensive and sophisticated treadmill, which has the effect of reducing the runner's gravity-related impact), 'performance' mattresses, which are designed to ease the runner's posture whilst asleep and so facilitate better quality sleep, as diverse options that may tweak a runner's performance. But the mental side is maybe where more gains are likely, albeit that this area is likely to be a long-term one for sports

scientists, rather than offering quick wins or shortcuts for runners or coaches.

Tim Noakes talks in his book *Lore of Running* of the Central Governor theory. In summary, this means that the reason why performance in endurance sport – in our case, running speed – declines as the muscles' level of lactate saturation increases, is because the brain tells the rest of the body that the level of exertion is reaching the level beyond which it may start damaging itself and not recover its former stable state at rest, or homeostasis. So, simplifying, slowing down because aerobically one is at a very high level of exertion is not a purely physical consequence, but happens because the brain makes it happen and we do not have a known mechanism by which the brain can avoid this. Unfortunately (or, on reflection, fortunately) there is not yet a sector within brain surgery that offers lobotomies as a surefire way to take chunks off your running PBs.

But applying this theory into practice, Noakes suggests that interval training has a role in moulding the Central Governor's tolerance of pain. What happens is that we work very hard for a fixed duration; recover in the interval; repeat the exertion again; recover again; and so on. This convinces the brain that with a combination of extreme hard work and suitable recovery we can extend our limits. Of course, races don't offer us the chance of a recuperative break, but one can understand how the brain can build up a tolerance on the basis that the level of discomfort has a finite duration that ends at the finish line.

Invariably, elite runners will speak of the importance of the brain, often in fairly simple ways. We should of course consider their views, but an elite athlete is just that; they are not necessarily sports psychologists, coaches or great thinkers. A British Olympic Champion said 'On the start line we are all the same physically. We've all done the same training and it's about who wants it most.' Well, yes and no. It's a nice sound bite about desire, self-belief and the winning mindset, but it does not bear up to rational scrutiny. In this champion's event, the 100m, the eight men on the start line will clearly have some physical differences – even the generalist TV viewer would be able to spot this, never mind the experienced sprints coach. This will affect

their start, their biomechanics and so on. And although their training will share many common aspects, there will also be some subtle differences that will surely be relevant in the range of their performances – say between 9.7 and 10.0 seconds in an Olympic final. That's 3 per cent. As one leading British high-performance sports consultant who has advised the UK funding agencies on the

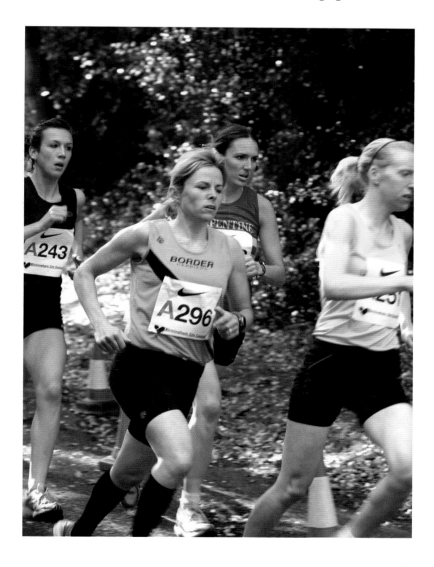

Racing around other runners can help your mind to focus on things other than increasing fatigue.

allocation of many millions of pounds into elite sports programmes, pithily stated, 'Elite athletes don't know what they don't know.'

However, it is notable that few runners below elite level really focus on the mental aspects of training and performance in the way they do the physical side of it, along with nutrition, conditioning and hydration. For example, the number of runners who will seek some professional sports nutrition advice will far exceed the number who ever invest in a sports psychologist. And it is fair to say that most coaches will have a similarly generalist approach to 'mental training'. So all in all, it's underutilized. We can therefore take a look at some pointers that may assist.

Having spent many hours listening to and talking to coaches and elite distance runners, they will often describe how efficiently they 'compartmentalize' their lives. That is, they are extremely focused and meticulous in all aspects of their training – and they do so separate from all other parts of their life. Thus for 2–3 hours a day they are athletes, but for the rest of it, although it is structured to assist high performance, they 'park' the mental focus on running and concentrate on work, children, domestics – whatever is needed to stay on top of things. For elite British woman Mara Yamauchi it has included polishing her Japanese language skills; for two-time Olympic marathon fourth-placer Jon Brown it has covered childcare and greyhound rearing. It is not clear if this focused time management is a learned skill that evolves as their running status increases or if it is something acquired at an early stage, but it is a common trait and one that many runners could benefit from.

In his excellent autobiography *From Last to First*, Charlie Spedding, Olympic Marathon medallist in 1984, talks about self-belief and goal-setting. His views correlate with the earlier comment about many runners not believing what they can aspire to if they put

the effort in. He describes how in his local north-east region a job was advertised with a £60,000 salary. The employers were mystified when nobody applied. They readvertised the exact same role, but offered only £25,000 and were inundated with applicants. Most of us will know or have met people in senior work roles whom we do not regard as being notably more competent, intelligent or skilled than ourselves – but what they have done is to believe what they can achieve and put themselves in a position to do so. In the running context, this is comparable to the many thousands of mid-packers who will marvel at the good club runners and just assume that their performances are always for 'other people', when in many cases the mid-pack could aspire to match these levels as long as they are prepared to do the groundwork.

Learning From the Elite – Applying Good Practice

It is not always clear how runners and coaches can learn from and apply what the elite do. From a human interest angle it can be fascinating to see what goes on 'behind the scenes' for a world-class runner when they aren't winning big races. This covers both the training and the 'rest of life' aspects. Indeed, once you have seen your first 100 elite athlete training plans, it is questionable what you will gain from studying the detail of elite runner 101, beyond any quirks about their lifestyle, other interests, diet and so on. However, for people right at the very top of the sport it is reasonable to accept that what they are doing represents best practice in terms of maximizing performance. Or, at least, very good practice.

As non-elite runners, you have to make certain judgements regarding what you understand to be best practice. It is extremely unlikely you will be able to copy it completely, even when building up to it gradually. To take an obvious example, if the elite runner covers an average of 115 miles per week, you probably will not be able to emulate this for reasons such as the elite runner will:

- have built up to this over many years;
- in all likelihood do most of this mileage on a softer surface than road, which you may not be able to replicate;
- probably not have another job, or will at most work part time, so will in all likelihood have far more hours in which to train;
- probably sleep about 10–11 hours per 24-hour cycle, either one long sleep at night or 8–9 hours at night plus a daily siesta between training sessions. This has substantial influence on what training load is sustainable;
- have regular – maybe even daily – massage to enable quicker recovery;
- have regular sport-specific medical back-up to ensure that training is being absorbed and is not leading to overtraining syndrome.

So you are extremely unlikely to be able to match this scenario. On the other hand, there may be some specifics of the training that you can repeat – albeit at your own relative speed – because they make good sense for your own circumstances and goals. For example:

- The elite runner may total about 100 miles for the five longest runs in a marathon build-up. If you are building up a good base of 13–15 milers in your general training, then this is the sort of load you could reasonably go for.
- The elite runner may as part of their half-marathon prep do a series of 5 × 9-minute reps at half-marathon pace, with a 2-minute easy run recovery. Can you do the same session? Yes, you can, though you do need to factor in that if the elite runner is a 61-minute half-marathoner and you are a 91-minute runner, the session at their half-marathon pace will be somewhat more intense for them than your reps at your half-marathon pace. To make the session more directly comparable, you might think about making your session 5 × 12 minutes at your half-marathon pace, so that you are covering a similar proportion of the race distance; or you could make the 5 × 9-minute reps at something between your 10km and 10-mile race pace – in effect, it would be your race pace that you could sustain in a 61-minute race, like the elite half-marathoner.

You will need to make similar judgement calls on other aspects of applying what elite athletes do, across areas such as: diet; strength and conditioning; alcohol; and planning. It is also not unknown for world-level runners to choose races that have a degree of trade-off between ideal long-term planning and financial reward.

KEY POINTS

- There are no magic or quick-fix training sessions.
- Harder training sessions have benefit in more than one aspect of improving performance.
- Plan your training in some detail and keep a record of what you do.
- The mental aspects of distance running performance are probably underutilized by most runners.
- Avoid any shortcuts in your general build-up phase, so that you are in the best shape to move on to the event specifics.

CHAPTER 4

MARATHON AND HALF-MARATHON TRAINING SPECIFICS

'To describe the agony of a marathon to some-one who's never run is like trying to explain colour to someone who was born blind.'

Jerome Drayton,
Canadian Marathon Record Holder

'Marathoning is like cutting yourself unexpect-edly. You dip into the pain so gradually that the damage is done before you are aware of it. Unfortunately, when awareness comes, it is excruciating.'

John Farrington,
Australian 2.11 marathoner and Olympian

'There is the truth about the marathon and very few of you have written the truth. Even if I explain to you, you'll never understand it, you're outside of it.'

Douglas Wakiihuri, World Marathon
Champion 1987 speaking to journalists

Marathon Essentials

The quotes above are all from marathon elites who have been there, often; done it, to an outstanding level; and worn the T-shirt, sweat-soaked, salt-encrusted and maybe bloodied round the nipples. The marathon, more than any other event in the running programme from 100m to 100km, is the one that captures modern runners' imaginations, whilst in many cases also often leaving them

ultimately disappointed at how they get to grips (or don't) with the event. If we can strip away some of the mystique and set out a few basics, that may help us with some specific and objective preparation for it:

- Its duration for the vast majority of readers of this book will be somewhere between, say, 2 hours 30 and 4 hours 30 minutes.
- It will be carried out with at least 99 per cent of the energy provided aerobically.
- Depending on your level of performance, you are likely to operate during a marathon at about 75–80 per cent of your VO_2 max and at about 80–90 per cent of your lactate threshold. Your training should not lose sight of this.
- Its duration is likely to be longer than any other sustained aerobic sport or exercise that runners may have done – with cycling and Ironman triathlons the possible exception for a few.
- It will usually take place on tarmac.
- Unlike all shorter running events, you are unlikely to cover the full marathon distance in a single training run, for reasons described below.
- The gruelling nature of the event means that if your target race goes worse than you had planned, you will need numerous weeks before you have another chance to race the distance again effectively, unlike other races further down the endurance

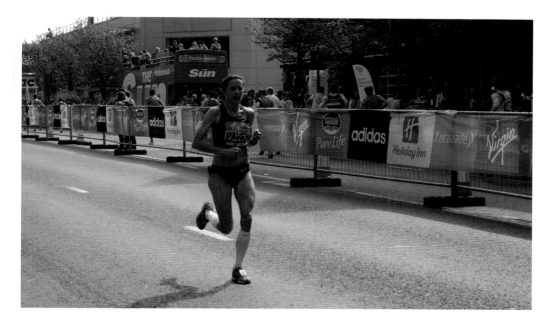

It is difficult even for the elite to hold form at the end of a marathon.

spectrum. This certainly affects the mental side of a marathon, both the training and the running of it on the big day.

- Unlike all shorter endurance events, including 20-mile races, your body cannot store enough glycogen to enable you to race the distance using only energy derived from carbohydrates. You have to train the body to run at a pace using fatty acids (of which we have an immense supply). The conversion of fatty acids to usable energy in the muscles has four times as many chemical processes as the production of the same amount of energy from carbohydrate.
- The long run does of course need to become longer. It also assumes a greater significance in the overall training plan. This starts to impact on training in the couple of days leading into and coming out of the long run.

Because the event is such a challenge, it is certainly a great feeling on those occasions when everything falls into place. Former British elite runner Paul Evans describes how when he won the Chicago Marathon in a PB of 2.08.52 there was a turn in the road at 22 miles where he could see the runners behind him. By this stage the pain was starting to build up, but he was still keeping a strong pace. He had enough mental agility remaining to do the maths and he knew that the chasing group could not find the change in pace to bridge the gap he had built up, so sure was he that the pace he could maintain for the remaining twenty minutes would be strong enough for the win. It's a great feeling that other runners can share, reaching a late stage of a marathon where mind and body work together to tell you that the combination of the remaining distance, your level of discom-

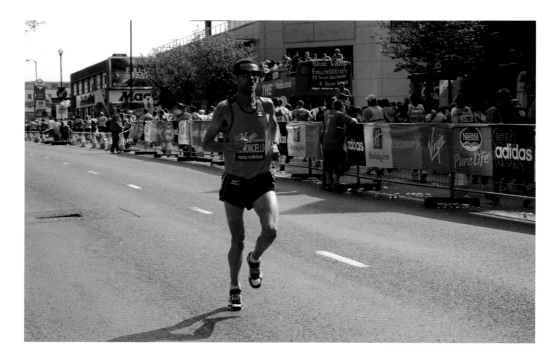

This elite runner keeps a good posture at the 22-mile point.

fort and what is shown on your watch add up to a job well done.

The Schedules

These carry on from where the general training plans have taken you in the previous three months. The progression is all about evolution, not revolution, so you won't wake up one Monday morning, on what is shown as Day 1 of the marathon-specific phase, as a different athletic specimen from the one who went to bed on the Sunday night a few hours earlier. And without wishing to labour the point, the better you have trained through the general phase, the more you can reap from the specific marathon phase.

There are two levels shown. At Level One, you are doing some purposeful training to ensure you are prepared to run the whole way round, with long runs up to 21 miles, and to make some inroads into training to improve 10km performances and underpin marathon progress. The more advanced level sits just below what we could call the full-on club runner, who is at that crossroads where certain lifestyle choices are planned and managed to fit around the running goals.

Do bear in mind that, particularly at less advanced levels, you may well improve your half-marathon – and indeed 10km – PB in races leading into your marathon. This is mainly because the marathon prep is probably the most thorough aerobic training you have yet carried out, so even without the 10km-specificity, the marathon training may hone you into better 10km shape.

Level One and Level Two Mileages

	Level One	Level Two
Average mileage for main eight-week block pre-taper	40	47
Total mileage of five longest runs	92	104
Maximum weekly mileage	45	54

Fat Burning Pace in the Marathon

Often misunderstood, perhaps the most emphatic and helpful summary of fat-burning pace is provided by global marathon coaching guru Renato Canova in his marathon brochure produced on behalf of the IAAF, the World Governing Body for athletics. When you run at about your lactate-threshold pace, you derive roughly 75 per cent of your energy from carbohydrate and 25 per cent from fatty (lipids) acid. When you run at about your aerobic threshold – which in elite runners is very close to their marathon pace – the proportions are much closer to 50 per cent carbohydrate and 50 per cent fatty acids. At shorter endurance races between 1,500 and 5,000m, your energy is provided almost entirely by carbohydrates. Whilst slowing the pace down to something gentler than marathon pace, you will use fatty acids as the source for most of the energy consumed.

Two key points emerge from this. First, the better you are trained so that your fastest running pace when using a higher percentage of fatty acids is close to your race pace when relying primarily on carbohydrates, the better prepared you are to 'convert' your half-marathon pace to a strong marathon result. Conversely, you have to ensure that during the marathon you avoid shifting too close to your lactate-threshold pace, or, whatever

carbo-loading you have done beforehand, and whatever you take on board during the race, you will run down your muscle glycogen at too early a stage to maintain the overzealous pace using exclusively fatty acids.

The schedules below have two particular types of repetition sessions, which, backed up of course by long runs to develop muscular endurance and some capacity to metabolize fatty acids at a steady speed, seem to be of benefit and may be different from what many readers have tried before. The two sessions are structured along the lines of:

- A bout of running at marathon pace *plus* some standard interval training of fairly short efforts at about 5km race pace, close to VO_2 max, to deplete muscle glycogen rapidly *plus* a further bout of running at marathon pace, to enable the runner to practise this pace in a relatively depleted state.
- Mid-length efforts (between 5 and 7 minutes) of between 10km pace and threshold pace, alternating between similar-length efforts at slightly slower than marathon pace. This teaches the body to shift slightly (that is, increase) the speed at which it is juggling the utilization of mainly glycogen with mainly fatty acids. The focus on these sessions, which should last between about 60 to maximum 90 minutes in order to balance a level of

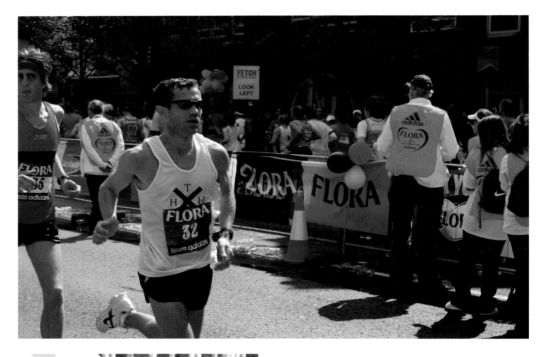

ABOVE: This experienced marathoner knows how to stay focused in the final miles.

BELOW: Metronomic even pace helped this runner to break 3 hours.

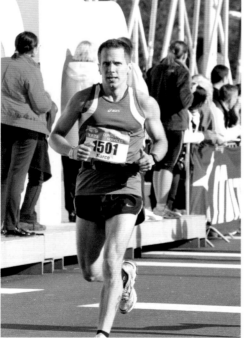

challenge with being right on the limits of what is manageable, is more about gradually pushing the pace of the slightly slower fat-burning efforts, and not so much about the pace of the faster stints.

Whilst emphasizing that there are no magic sessions or shortcuts, and of course there is more than one way to skin the long-distance cat, these sessions seem to be very effective in helping well-trained and sensible runners to optimize their marathon performances in the context of their 10km and half-marathon times.

The Taper

The earlier comments regarding needing about ten to twelve days to go through the adaptation and super-compensation process of training are in line with the requirements of a marathon taper – which, remember, will usually be quoted in multiples of seven days because that it is how most training is structured, not because the body actually operates on this weekly timescale. So it is not uncommon to do a final hard specific session about eleven to twelve days before the marathon, even though this is within the tapering phase.

You need to keep the balance between gradually winding down from the training peak and avoiding any detraining – so this is definitely not a full fortnight of putting your feet up or even casual jogging. That can be considered after the marathon. You may have read of tapers of three or even four weeks at elite level. These will invariably be for runners on the very limits of high mileage, maybe 130–150 per week, so they may take a week or two whereby they scale back to 'only' about 90–100 miles before a more pronounced reduction.

The most effective tapers tend to use a reduction in volume of about 30–35 per cent in the penultimate week and then a further 30 per cent or so in the final week. Of course, the final week's mileage will vary depending on whether you include or omit the small matter of the marathon itself. An amusing but useful anecdote on the final taper week is offered by Paul Evans again, who, jestingly referring to his initial aborted marathons, said his final week's mileage was 'about 20, including the race!'

In general, the last ten to twelve days are about keeping in touch with the sort of harder training paces you have been developing over weeks and months, but not stretching the envelope as far as fatiguing yourself at these paces. So, just because the sessions are reduced in volume/duration, do not feel the need to run them quicker than the suggested paces; instead, you should be finishing the sessions at about the point where fatigue starts to creep in.

The last three or four days should be very minimal running – and you should definitely not be looking to deploy the freed-up energy and time into any further training activities. Avoid new forays into stretching, strength and conditioning, or aerobic cross-training at this late stage. Any training options not taken on board in the previous months are not going to be of marathoning benefit now.

Guiding Principles

- If you miss a hard session, do not piggyback it either the day before or day after another hard session.
- If you do not yet have a record of 3km or 5km races, don't agonize excessively over exact 3km or 5km pace in the interval sessions. But do gauge the pace so that it is about 20–30 seconds per mile quicker than a 10km race pace, although not so much quicker that you can't sustain it, fairly evenly, for the duration of the interval session.
- If you are training for a flat marathon, do ensure that some of your longest runs are on similarly flat terrain, as you want to practise that precision and evenness of effort that the race will require. But earlier on in the 13-week programme it is fine to include some hills in the longer runs.
- Treat strength and conditioning as an integral part of the training rather than as a casual add-on, but do not treat it as a replacement for the running elements. You will see that strength and conditioning are focused more towards the earlier

parts of the programme, on the rationale that once you get into the heaviest running volume the energy and time available may be at its tightest, so conditioning should have been topped up already to get you through this period.

- Running at marathon pace (MP). This is assuming a flat stretch of good-quality tarmac; cool, windless weather; light-weight racing kit; a tapered fully hydrated runner; high (but controlled) adrenalin. In practice, once you deviate from this ideal scenario, you will invariably run slightly slower than what you perceive, and what your heart-rate monitor may show, to be marathon effort. Experience suggests that a typical marathon effort in training will be about 10–15 seconds per mile slower than target MP.

- Different race paces. A reasonable guideline for runners with a good base of endurance training is 'double the race distance and add 20 seconds per mile'. The distance where the majority of runners do not make this sort of conversion is between half-marathon and marathon.

Some Final Tips

The Day Before

- Think positive – don't agonize over any training missed through illness/injury/bad weather/lifestyle commitments, but instead look back at what you have done – there will be some good long runs of 20 miles and more; some races; some sustained efforts at marathon pace; some rep sessions – all good event-specific preparation.

- Make sure you have understood all the race day transport and logistic arrangements, and especially if it's a big city event where you need to allow extra time for moving in a large crowd.

- Try to avoid getting too involved in friends' and family's spectating plans, beyond some basic courtesies. It can become draining working out everybody's timetables whilst pinning down your own plans.

- A unit or two (maximum) of alcohol the night before will not harm performance the next day as long as you hydrate accordingly, and if this is your usual intake and may help you get to sleep, then no worries.

- Unless you feel particularly sleepy, an unduly early night is not a necessity as you will be more likely to lie awake, unable to sleep. Wait until you feel sleepy before going to bed. A slightly curtailed single night's sleep will not affect your performance the next morning.

On the Day

- Have breakfast between 2 and 3½ hours before start time – by now you should know what works regards timing, digestion, hunger pangs, amount and specific type of food. Ensure that there is familiar food if you are away at a hotel – if in doubt, bring the basics with you.

- Fluids – keep topped up, about 200ml/⅓ of a pint each 30 minutes up to the last 30/45 minutes before the start.

- Warm up – if space allows, do a 3–5 minutes' jog about 20 minutes beforehand – at a slow pace this will help make MP feel easier to start with and will not impact on glycogen depletion; the slow pace will be fuelled almost entirely by fat and we all have ample supplies.

- Once stripped off, if weather is cool/cold have a bin liner and/or old T-shirt that can be discarded once the gun goes, just to keep the muscles warmish.

- Double-knot your shoelaces – you do not want to lose time or break stride for an oversight like this.

Once the Gun Goes

- Don't worry about time lost at the start if you not cannot get into proper pace for the first kilometre/mile; you will gradually claw this back, assuming you are starting in a zone with broadly similar-pace runners.
- Do try to relax and enjoy the first hour or so, as long as you keep to an even pace. It will not be possible to concentrate intensely on the running for 3 hours or more, so make the most of the scenery early on because at 23 miles it's unlikely you'll be able to be so relaxed.
- Typically, a very well-paced run may lose about 90 seconds in the second half of the race, but almost all of this should be in the last 4 miles. Your 20-mile split should be very close to simply two times your 10-mile split — if you are slowing slightly from 16/17 miles then you will in all likelihood slow more markedly from 21/22 onwards.
- Do start drinking early — take on approx. 200ml every 5km from about 8–10km. Many find that alternating water with a carbo/sports drink/gel is the right balance.
- Also take on sponges and douse the head and shoulders with water if available.
- Avoid any surges, whatever bursts of cheering you encounter, or inspirational landmarks or training rivals or friends you pass — this will run down your glycogen faster than you want.
- Follow the blue line or shortest marked route as closely as you can.
- Bear in mind the 'talking test' — you should be comfortable to talk at 13 miles and ideally to about 15–16 miles. If not, you have probably set out too fast.

Analysing the Final Result

If you have set or agreed an upper realistic target based on ideal weather, sensible pacing and everything going just right on the day, if you finish within 2–3 minutes of this time you should be pleased with a great run. Any target less than 2 × (½ marathon time × 1.06) is unlikely to be realistic. If you finish between about 4–6 minutes of your ideal target, that is still a very solid run over a very hard and unpredictable event. If you are more than 7 minutes slower than your target, you should be able to identify at least one element in your training, overall preparation and how you handled the event on the day that can be improved upon next time round (assuming there will be a next time).

A Level Two 'Graduate'

An athlete the author has coached for over three years has trained broadly to the volume, structure and periodization of the programme above. Now aged forty, she was a reasonable level club and university runner, fitting her running, conditioning and races around raising three young children and a full-time job in senior financial management. Over the three years of training she has progressed from a 42-minute 10km level down to 38.20 and improved her half-marathon PB to 83 minutes. In April 2011 she made her marathon debut in London, clocking a satisfying 3 hours 10 minutes. She slightly raised the training level through the summer and was delighted to run a 2 hours 58 minutes marathon in October 2011.

What this anecdote does not capture is her extremely high level of motivation and single-minded time-management ability. Nor does the schedule build in the factor that in early March, taking drastic action to avoid a dog, she broke her elbow and had a substantially reduced running programme at a key training phase. Her conditioning and strength training were probably just as important as the running training in her progress, because by keeping various niggles at bay there were no long runs or harder sessions that needed to

Level One Training Programme

Day	Week 1 40 Miles	Week 2 37 Miles	Week 3 29 Miles	Week 4 39 Miles	Week 5 36 Miles	Week 6 (Biggest Week) – 45 Miles
1			Strength and conditioning	40min easy		
2	10min w/up – 4 × (6min at 10km pace/6 min at MP + 20sec per mile) – 1 mile w/d	40 min easy	w/up – 15min at MP (90sec) – 6 × 2min at 3/5km pace (90sec jog) – 15min at MP 5min easy	60min easy inc 8 × 20sec strides	10–15min w/up – 10 × 2.5min at c.5km pace (90sec) – w/down	10min w/up – 5 × (5.5min at 10km pace/5.5 min at MP + 20sec per mile) – 5min easy
3	40min easy	60min easy/steady inc 8 × 15–20sec strides		10min easy – 5 × (5min at 10km pace/5min at MP + 20sec per mile) – w/down	40min easy	40min easy
4	15min easy 60min at MP – 5min easy	1 mile easy – 20min at MP (90sec) – 10 × 90sec at 3k/5k pace (60sec) – (90sec) 15min at MP – 5min jog – quite long session in all	10min easy – 35min at MP – 5min easy	Strength and conditioning	10min w/up reps at c.10–mile pace – 14–12–10 9min (2min jog after each) – 1 mile easy	1 mile easy – 75min at MP – 5min easy
5	Strength and conditioning	Strength and conditioning			Stength and conditioning	
6				18 miles easy/steady – MP + 45/50 sec per mile		
7	16 miles steady 2 hr 20/2hr 25 max at MP + 40sec per mile	16 miles progressive e.g. 3 miles easy – 9 miles at MP + 35/40sec per mile – 4 miles at MP + 10sec per mile	Half-Marathon race		16 miles progressive e.g. 3 miles easy – MP + 60/70sec – 7 miles at MP + 30/35sec – 6 miles at MP + 10sec per mile	21 miles steady or max of 3hr

Day	Week 7 40 Miles	Week 8 43 Miles	Week 9 29 Miles Ease into Half-Marathon	Week 10 33 Miles	Week 11 34 Miles	Week 12 28 Miles	Week 13 38 Miles Miles inc Marathon
1							
2	w/up – 20 min at MP (90sec) – 10 × 90sec at 3km/5km pace (60sec) – (90sec) – 20min at MP – 5min jog	10–15min w/up –7 × 4.5min at c.5km pace (2min jog) – w/down	10min easy – 5 × 6min at c.10km pace (80sec jog) – w/down	40min easy	40min easy including 8 × 20sec strides	10min easy – 8 × 6.5 min at 10 mile pace (70sec jog) – w/down	10–15min w/up – 4 × 3.5min at 5km pace (90sec jog) – w/down
3	Strength and conditioning	40min easy	30min easy	60min steady	10min w/up – 5 × (6min at 10km pace/7min at MP + 20 sec per mile) – 5min easy	30min easy	25min easy
4	10min easy – 4 × 12min at slightly slower than 10km pace (2min) – w/down	1 mile easy – 80min at c.MP – 5min easy	1 mile easy – 30min at MP – 5min easy	10min easy – 2 sets of 7 × 80sec at c.3km pace (40 sec jog/3min jog between sets) – w/down		10min easy – 20min at c.10km pace or a touch slower – 10min easy	15min easy – 2km at MP – 5min easy
5		Strength and conditioning			w/up – 2 sets 7 × 60sec at controlled 3km pace (40sec recovery/ 3min jog between sets) – w/down		
6	40min steady						
7	17 miles progressive 2 miles easy + MP + 60/70 sec – 8 miles at MP + 30/35 sec – 7 miles at MP + 10sec per mile	20 miles steady, good pace, MP + 30sec per mile	Half-Marathon race	1 mile easy – 16 miles at MP+ 10/15sec per mile	1 mile easy/ 13 miles at c.MP – 5 min easy	1 mile easy – 8 miles at c.MP + 10sec per mile – 5 min easy; use similar terrain to marathon course if possible	Marathon

Level Two Training Programme

Day	Week 1 46 Miles	Week 2 39 Miles	Week 3 (Easier Week) 32 Miles	Week 4 43 Miles	Week 5 45 Miles	Week 6 (Biggest Week) 54 Miles	Week 7 49 Miles
1	45min steady inc 8 × 20sec strides		Strength and conditioning			10min w/up – 5 × (6min at 10km pace/7min at MP + 15/20sec per mile) – 5min easy)	w/up – 25 min at MP (90sec at 3km/5km pace (60sec) – (90sec) – 20min at MP – 5min jog
2	10min w/up – 4 × (6min at 10km pace/ 7min at MP + 30sec per mile) – 1 mile w/d	35min easy	w/up – 5 × (6min at 10km pace/ 6min at MP + 30sec per mile	45min easy	10–15min w/up –9 × 3 min at c.5km pace (90sec jog) then 30 min at MP – w/down	40min easy	40min easy
3	40min easy	60min easy/ steady inc 8 × 15–20 sec strides		60min easy inc 8 × 20 sec strides	30min easy	1 mile easy – 75min at MP	10min easy – 4 × 13min at slightly slower than 10km pace (2min) – w/down
4	1 mile easy – 65min at MP + 10sec per mile – 5min easy	1 mile easy – 20min at MP (90sec) – 12 × 90sec at 3km/ 5km race pace (60sec) – (90 sec) – 15min at MP – 5min jog – long session in all	10min easy – 30min at MP – 5min easy	10min easy 25min at MP (90sec) –8 × 2min at 5km race pace (60sec) – (90sec) – 20min at MP – w/down	10min w/up reps at c.10 mile pace –14 –12–10–9min (2min after each) – 1mile (easy)	45min easy	Strength and conditioning
5	Strength and conditioning	Strength and conditioning	30min easy inc 1 × 4 at half marathon pace	Strength and conditioning	Strength and conditioning		40min steady
6					45min steady	22/23 miles steady – MP + 45/50sec per mile or 3hr/ 3hr 10max	19 miles progressive, 2 miles easy – MP + 60/ 70sec – 9 miles at MP + 30/35sec – 8 miles at MP + 10sec per mile

Day	Week 1	Week 2	Week 3	Week 4	Week 5
7	17 miles steady or 2hr 20/2hr 25 max	17 miles progressive e.g. 3 miles easy – 9 miles at MP + 35/40 sec per mile – 5 miles at MP + 10sec per mile	half-marathon race	20 miles easy/steady – MP + 60/70 sec – per mile or 2hours 50 max	19 miles progressive e.g. 3 miles easy – MP + 60/70sec – 9 miles at MP + 30/35sec – 7 miles at MP + 10sec per mile

Day	Week 8 49 Miles	Week 9 33 Miles Ease into Half Marathon	Week 10 46 Miles	Week 11 45 Miles	Week 12 30 Miles	Week 13 39 Miles inc Marathon
1						
2	10–15min w/up – 7 × 4 min at c.5km pace (2min jog) – w/down	30min easy	40min easy	50min easy inc 8 × 20sec strides	10min easy – 8 × 6.5min at 10 mile pace (70sec jog) – w/down	10–15min w/up – 4 × 3.5 min at 5km pace (90sec jog) – w/down
3	40min easy	1 mile easy – 30min at MP – 5min easy	60min steady	10min w/up – 6 × (6min at 10km pace/ 7min at MP + 20sec per mile) – 5min easy	40min easy	25min easy
4	1 mile easy – 80min at c.MP – 5min easy	30min easy inc 1 × 4min at half-marathon pace	10min easy – 10 × 2min at c.3km/5km pace (75sec jog/90sec jog) – 40min at target MP	50min easy	10min easy – 25min at c. 10km pace – 10min easy	15min easy – 2km at MP – 5min easy
5	Strength and conditioning		45min easy	w/up – 12 × 90sec at controlled 3km/5km pace (60sec jog) – w/down		
6	40min easy inc 8 × 20sec strides					
7	21–22 miles steady/MP + 45sec per mile or max 3hr	half-marathon race	1 mile easy – 18 miles at MP+ 10–15 sec per mile	1 mile easy/13 miles at c.MP 5min easy	1 mile easy – 9 miles at c.MP + 10sec per mile – 5min easy; use similar terrain to marathon course if possible	marathon

be missed or compromised to protect any low-level injury.

And If That's Not Enough ...

The above level two has a total of 490-odd miles in the eleven weeks before a taper, or an average of 45 miles per week. In terms of actual running time it is a weekly commitment of about six or seven hours depending on your pace. Also, of course, there is a spin-off on other parts of your life from doing so, plus additional time spent on any conditioning and stretching. If you wish to push the boat out further, maybe having done one or two cycles of this schedule, then think about the following principles to add an extra challenge:

- Look to extend the steady and easy runs towards 60 minutes, as there will be extra aerobic adaptations, albeit slight at this pace, in the final minutes of the run.
- Look to add a sixth weekly run, either weekly or fortnightly, and use a duration and pace that takes into account the previous bullet point.
- Not losing sight of the point below about a cautious approach to long runs too close to the full marathon distance, consider extending the runs shown in the schedule in the 13–16-mile range towards the 16–18-mile range. You need to be pragmatic about assessing how this impacts on your body the following day or two. You can gradually get used to the longer distance, but regular 18-milers at a solid pace will always take some toll the next day.

Things to avoid doing at this next level would include:

- Extending the long run any closer to the full marathon distance than about 24–25 miles as an absolute maximum. Even at elite level there is some caution about going the full distance or over-distance in training. In summary, these extra miles give a level of depletion that weakens the immune system, leaving you vulnerable to infection for about 36–48 hours however well you refuel after the run. Also the sheer distance will require extra days of recovery into the following week, compromising other purposeful specific sessions. Also – in the context of weekly mileage in the mid- to high forties – doing somewhat more than half the volume in one single run, for a marathon target, is pushing the muscles, joints and tendons beyond a distance that the rest of the week's training has prepared them for.
- Extending warm-up and warm-down runs just to add mileage into the diary. Once you have achieved the purpose of warming up or warming down, you have achieved it and there is no benefit in doing further at a very easy pace.
- Adding extra reps to the interval sessions (well, it might just be a temptation, although practical coaching experience indicates it's not what most runners fancy doing once the designated number of reps is completed). If you are accurately doing the session at something like 3km pace, a combination of logic and physiology should indicate that there is a limited volume/distance that is manageable at this pace, within the structure of effort versus recovery. Adding volume must mean a slower average pace for the session and therefore a lesser amount of running done at the target pace.
- Avoid adding double runs until you have reached a ceiling at what seems manageable and beneficial on a single-run basis. There is not an exact number at which

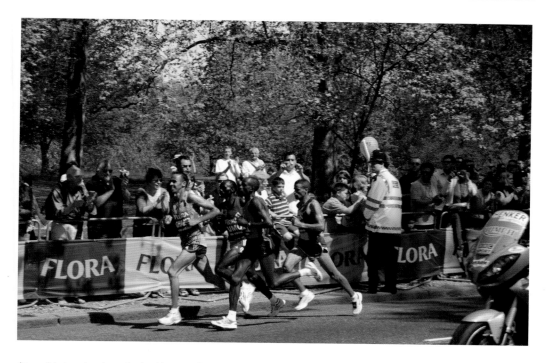

At world-class level you find athletes still racing fast through the twenty-sixth mile.

'doubling' starts to make sense, but bear in mind that it would be a higher weekly mileage for marathon runners – or indeed half-marathoners – than for 1,500m types. Something in the region of 60–65 miles a week would be about the volume to start adding that small aerobic benefit that occasional doubles might bring. Realistically, occasional double days start at a performance level where the majority of readers of this book are unlikely to go.

Advanced Runner Case Histories

As an example of how this all may work, here are some training samples of a female athlete

coached by the author for the five years from summer 2003. The training plans show two weeks from her general phase, sixteen to eighteen weeks before a marathon, and two weeks from her specific build-up, six to seven weeks before the race.

As background, she had a reasonable level of ability but was not unusually gifted. Her debut 10km after about six months of training to a reasonable volume of 45 miles per week and with a sensible structure was achieved in 44 minutes. She was born in 1970 so the five-year window summarized below is arguably when she was at her physical peak for long-distance running.

She worked mainly from home in London during this period, in the museum sector. She made approximate fortnightly trips to north

Female Runner – General Endurance Phase

1	50min easy inc 8 × 20sec strides
2	w/up – group session at track, e.g. 6 or 7 × 1,200m at 5km race pace with between 1.5–2min jog
3	am 30min easy; pm 45min easy to steady
4	60–65min steady
5	50min easy
6	w/up – 4 × 10min at approximate 10-mile race pace (2min jog recovery) – w/down
7	15 miles steady
Total	67 miles
8	50min easy inc 8 × 2-second strides
9	w/up – Group session at track e.g. 8min at 10-mile pace (90sec jog) – 8 × 600m at 3km race pace (60/70sec jog) – 8min at 10-mile pace – w/down. On a fortnightly cycle the Tuesday sessions would avoid repeating the same paces in successive weeks
10	55min easy
11	60/65min steady
12	rest
13	w/up – hill reps e.g. 3 sets of 6 × 25/30sec climb, off-road surface, jog back recovery and about 2–3min easy run between each set of 6 reps – w/down
14	15 miles steady – the distance would vary between 13 and maximum 17 miles
Total	52 miles

Scotland to her employer's HQ and was able to plan her training around these occasional but demanding travel commitments. She is married to another good club-level distance runner.

In the first year in which she broke 2.50 for the marathon she ranked twentieth in Britain at the distance. On the one hand that's a fine achievement given the many, many thousands of women who complete the distance each year, and winning a marathon that is officially graded by the World Governing Body as a second-tier race (behind the real big hitters such as London, New York, Paris et al.) is immensely satisfying. On the other hand, it is almost exactly 1 minute per mile behind real world-class level and is equivalent to a male running about 2.28. The author believes that at any time there are scores of women involved in marathoning in the UK who could reach this sort of level given time, commitment and a structured programme.

Her other PBs came down to 18.05 5km/36.31 10km; 60 minutes for 10 miles; and 79.02 for the half-marathon. What is interesting is that anyone with these PBs should be able to train to run a 2.49 marathon (or indeed, a couple of minutes quicker), but so few, male or female, manage to do so.

Female Runner – Marathon-Specific Phase

1	50min easy inc 8 × 20sec strides
2	w/up – group session at track, e.g. 6 × 1,500m or 1 mile at 10km race pace (60–70sec jog recovery) – w/down
3	am 30min easy; pm 45min easy to steady
4	90min steady
5	55/60min easy
6	am w/up – long reps at half-marathon pace e.g. 3 × 16–18min, 2.5 min jog recovery; pm 30min easy
7	19 miles progressive e.g. 3 miles easy/11 miles at about MP + 30–40sec per mile/5 miles at MP + 10–15sec per mile
Total	77 miles
8	50 min easy inc 8 × 2sec strides
9	w/up – Group session at track e.g. 9min at 10-mile pace (90sec jog) – 8 × 800m at 5km race pace (80sec jog) – 9min at 10-mile pace – w/down. On a fortnightly cycle the Tuesday sessions would avoid repeating the same paces in successive weeks
10	55/60min easy
11	am 30min easy; pm 60/65 steady
12	rest
13	w/up – 70–75min at target MP, on flat route
14	21/22 miles steady state at about MP + 45sec per mile
Total	75 miles

The first seven marathons listed on the right each represented a new PB, and the eighth was just a few seconds shy of her 2.49 PB. That's a good level of consistency in what is a notoriously unpredictable event. Every race was held on a flat, fast course and apart from two that were in slightly warm weather, all were held in good conditions for marathons.

The progression rate in the table is maybe the sort of rate of diminishing returns that seasoned runners can expect. Very roughly, from when the author started coaching this runner in Autumn 2003, she added maybe 15–20 per cent to her weekly mileage over

Female Runner – List of Marathons

2003	3.13 London
2004	2.59 London; 2.56 Abingdon (first)
2005	2.56 London; 2.52 Holland
2006	2.51 Edinburgh (first); 2.49 San Sebastian (first)
2007	2.49 London
2008	2.50 London (very warm conditions; possibly her best performance)

the following four to five years, a significant amount of higher-intensity running, a greater attention to detail in strength and conditioning, and logged up about a further 15,000 miles of training and racing. She achieved an improvement of about 20 minutes in the marathon and about 8 minutes over the half-marathon – that's around 10 per cent.

For a second case history we use Darren, from West London, 35 years old in 2011, and self-coached through his senior running days. Although he shares some character traits with all committed long-distance runners – those of single-mindedness, work ethic and good planning – he is perhaps in some ways more obsessive and driven than most, so he has ploughed himself into his work as an IT specialist. He does nothing by halves – except for half-marathons of course.

After some schoolboy enthusiasm for athletics in general, but no particular endurance focus, Darren let things slip in his early working years in the IT sector. By age twenty-five, his weight had soared to 14st 12lb (95kg).

He started training in April 2005 for his first marathon in Berlin in September 2005, achieving 3:08, weighing close to 13 stone (83kg). He then progressed through: April 2006, 2:51 (Boston); October 2006, 2:37 (Chicago); November 2006, 2:53 (New York City); April 2007, 2:41 (London); December 2008, 2:29 (Fukuoka); and October 2009, 2:34 (Dublin).

It is fair to say that Darren has slightly more basic endurance talent than the average person, because to advance from an overweight jogger to a 3.08 marathoner so quickly and then to push on to a 2.29 marathon in fewer than four years is fairly quick progress. However, in the following three years he did not manage to improve his PBs despite continuing with a heavy duty structured training programme and to a considerable degree building his non-working life around his running ambitions – which suggests that his talent is not in the highest echelons.

However, he bounced back in September 2011, clocking 2.29.45 in the Berlin Marathon, in the race where the world record was improved to 2.03.36. Darren actually rates the Berlin result as his best of all, even though he fell an agonizing 3 seconds short of his PB. His build-up had been carried out during a period of extremely long working hours and he was always struggling to keep a range of hip and lower leg niggles at bay, although the training volume and intensity were adhered to as planned. The Fukuoka (Japan) venue of his 2.29 tells you something about his mental focus. This is an iconic event in a nation where marathon running is the main national sport. Darren – with no ability in the Japanese language – sorted out all his own entry, travel and accommodation details in a race, which, bar a scant handful of international elite invitees, is a purely domestic affair in early December. With that 2.30 time as a major benchmark of marathon prowess, Darren had to dig in deeply as his mile splits slowed in the final stages. We won't quote his Anglo-Saxon exhortations in what may be a book for all the family, but the summary would be that he really did not want to go to all the trouble of preparing for the race, travelling at considerable expense, only to return home having run the 'wrong' side of 2.30.

If we look at extracts of his training, shown below, we see the sort of progression in form that most experienced runners would be very pleased to match over such a relatively short period. As he is a case study of one, we cannot quantify how much of this is due to innate ability and how much to a perfectly structured programme – or indeed how much extra bloody mindedness he found in the last hard stage on the Japanese tarmac. But the sort of specificity he evolved in his training in this phase should be seen as very good practice based on the outcome.

These two fortnightly extracts from Darren's general phase and from his Berlin 2011 build-up are worth considering, although the mileage totals will be more than most runners would be likely to cover and

nobody would wish to emulate the nagging sore adductors that had to be nursed through the training. Key points to note are:

- Flexibility, in that by virtue of his self-employed status he could arrange a key midweek long run.
- He's not a slave to mileage for its own

Two Extracts from Darren's Build-Up

Week Ending 20 March – 85 miles

M   8 miles easy at 7.30 miling

T   am 5 miles easy at 8 min pace; pm w/up – 5 × 2km at 10km race pace (2min jog) – w/down

W   am weights; pm 10 miles easy at 7.15

T   6 miles easy at 7.30 pace; pm w/up – 4 × 3km at 10km pace (2.5min jog) – w/down

F   8 miles easy at 7.30 miling

S   w/up – 5km park run at threshold then 4 × 1 mile cross-country hilly loops at about threshold (1min jog) – w/down

S   long run – 20 miles steady at 7.00 per mile

Week Ending 27 March – 74 miles

M   6 miles easy at 7.30 pace

T   am 6 miles easy at 7.50; pm w/up – 5 × 2km at 10km race pace (2min jog) – w/down. Reps 5sec quicker than same session 7 days prior, actually slightly quicker than sustainable 10km race pace

W   am weights; pm 8 miles at 7.15 pace

T   am 6 miles easy at 7.40pm; w/up 3 × 3km at 10km pace (2.5min jog) – w/down

F   7 miles easy at 7.30 pace

S   w/up – 5 mile flat road race 27.23, disappointing, one-paced, so couldn't hold pace after a quicker first mile – w/down

S   am 4 miles easy; pm w/up – road relay for club, 5 miles in 26.5, then 6 miles easy

---

Week Ending 14 August
(Berlin Minus 6 Weeks) – 104 Miles

M   8 miles easy at 8min miles; pm 8 miles easy at 7.30 miles

T   long run of 23 miles in 2.44. Average 7.08, but last 5 miles average 6.20 per mile

W   rest

T   am 8 miles easy at 8min miles; pm 2-mile w/up – 4 × 3km on treadmill at threshold pace (slightly slower than 10km race pace), 2min jog recovery – 1 mile w/down

F   am 8 miles easy at 7.30 miles; pm 8 miles easy at 7.15 miles

S   10 miles easy at 7.15 pace

S   Salisbury 30km – undulating and done at close to marathon effort

---

Week Ending 21 August – (Berlin Minus 5 Weeks) – 64 Miles

M   rest

T   rest – adductor sore

W   rest – adductor sore

T   am 8 miles easy at 7.40 miling; pm 8 miles steadier at 7.00 per mile to test adductors

F   am 8 miles easy at 7.30 pace; pm 8 miles easy at 7.30 pace

S   2 miles w/up – 10km race at 95% effort in 34.30, 1 mile w/down, disappointing results in terms of effort

S   7 miles easy – Burnham Beeches half-marathon at marathon effort in 77.15 – 3 miles easy. Encouraging result given the course and the managed level of effort

---

sake. Clearly, there is a lot of running week in, week out, but there are rest days and shorter, easier days so the principle of recovery is built in.

- Weights/conditioning are built into the pre-marathon phase when there is greater capacity of time and 'spare' energy.
- Shorter races are in the general training phase.
- A specific point for runners doing early autumn marathons such as Berlin or

Nottingham is that the choice of build-up races without a long journey can be somewhat limited, so Darren chose a couple of tough hilly races in the knowledge that the marathon effort could broadly be replicated, albeit the race pace would not be as swift as he could sustain on the long, flat avenues of Berlin.

- The faster training in the marathon build-up is actually not that fast, because he was honing in more on marathon pace. This is in contrast with the sessions in the late spring, when he was doing slightly shorter efforts at close to his maximum aerobic speed (vVO_2 max). This emphasizes the longer-term periodized nature of his build-up.

- A similar longer-term principle is shown in his long runs. The general build-up was about covering the distance at a relatively comfortable pace, whereas as the marathon approached the pace became more important.

Half-Marathon Schedule

Now that we have covered in detail the general training and some marathon specifics, the half-marathon specifics fall somewhere between the two. For most readers, the half-marathon target is likely to be between 80 minutes and 2 hours, or slightly over. So it is a pace not far short of the lactate threshold, but somewhat quicker than the marathon pace. It is a pace where, crucially, muscle glycogen will not be exhausted over the distance, so those very long marathon runs that train the fat-burning capacity become less relevant.

Given that the general training phase develops so much of the training base that

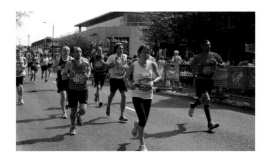

Make smart choices on marathon clothing to avoid overdressing in mild temperatures.

will apply to your half-marathon performance, there is less need for a full thirteen-week build-up after the general phase. Instead, two levels of a seven-week schedule are shown below. The main progressions from the general phase are:

- Slight increase in the long run so that the distance itself becomes less of a challenge.
- Building up the pace of parts of the longer runs to help you to balance speed and distance.
- A race at 10km or 10 miles to help to inform the target pace your half-marathon should aim for.
- More specific sessions at close to half-marathon pace.

Readers should be aware that from the coach's perspective in writing these schedules there is a challenge in making them 'fit for all'. A 70-minute half-marathon runner – and most years there are a couple of hundred in the UK – is running the distance at very close to their threshold pace, whereas the runner taking, say, 2 hours 15 minutes (and there will be many more of these than there are 70-minute whippets) is heading more towards the energy demands of an elite marathoner in terms of the balance of glycogen and fatty acid consumption. That said, most readers will fall into the middle ground at which these schedules are pitched.

Marathon Pace Predictors and Pacing

There are numerous tables on the Internet and in magazines that will convert race performances at other shorter distances to what they are 'worth' in a marathon. In general, these guidelines are fairly sensible, given certain caveats that are the runner's

Level One Seven-Week Schedule

	Week 1	Week 2	Week 3	Week 4	Week 5	Week 6	Week 7
Day 1	40min easy inc 6 × 20sec strides	40min easy inc 6 × 20sec strides	30min easy inc 6 × 20sec strides	35min very easy	45min easy inc 6 × 20sec strides	45min easy inc 6 × 20sec strides	30min easy inc 6 × 20sec strides
Day 2	w/up – 2 × 6 min at 10km pace (60sec recovery) + 7 × 2min at c.3km pace (80sec recovery) – w/down	w/up – 8 c.3.5min at 5km race pace (2min jog) – w/down	w/up – 6 × 8min at half-marathon pace (90sec recovery)	60min easy	w/up – 8 × 5min at between 10km and 10 mile race pace (60sec jog) – w/down	w/up – 50min progressive run, 35min at half marathon pace, 15min at 10k pace, w/down	w/up – 2 × 10min at half-marathon pace (90sec jog) + 1 × 5min at c.5km race pace – w/down
Day 3							30min easy
Day 4	w/up – 5 × 9 min at half-marathon race pace (90sec jog)	w/up 35min at half-marathon pace + 20sec per mile then 15min at half-marathon pace	35min steady	w/up – 10 × 2 min at 3km race pace (70sec jog) – w/down	w/up – 10min at half-marathon pace (60sec jog) – 5 × 2min at 5km race pace (60sec jog)	w/up – 10min at half marathon pace (90sec jog) – 3 × 4min at 5k race pace (2min jog) – w/down	
Day 5							
Day 6	15 miles steady	15 miles steady		15 miles progressive so, e.g. 3 miles easy, 7 miles at half-marathon pace + 40sec per mile, last 5 miles at approx half-marathon pace + 20/30 sec per mile	1 mile easy – 6 miles at half-marathon pace + c.30 sec per mile – 4 miles at half-marathon pace + 10sec per mile	1 mile easy – 8 miles at half marathon pace + 10sec per mile	
Day 7			10km or 10-mile race				Half-marathon race
Total miles	34	33	26	31	34	29	27

Level Two Seven-Week Schedule

	Week 1	Week 2	Week 3	Week 4	Week 5	Week 6	Week 7
Day 1	45min easy inc 6 × 20sec strides	45min easy inc 6 × 20sec strides	35min easy inc 6 × 20sec strides	30min easy	45min easy inc 6 × 20sec strides	45min easy inc 6 × 20sec strides	30min easy inc 6 × 20sec strides
Day 2	w/up – 3 × 6min at 10km pace (60 sec jog) + 10 × 90 sec at 3km race pace (60sec jog) – w/down	w/up – 2 sets of 5 × 3min at 5km pace (80sec jog and 3min jog between sets – w/down	w/up – 6 × 9 min at half-marathon pace (90sec jog) – w/down	60min easy inc 8 × 20sec strides	w/up – 4 × 14 min at half-marathon pace (2.5min jog)	w/up – 8 × 6 min between 10km and 10-mile race pace (60sec jog)	w/up – 2 × 6min at 10km race pace (90sec recovery) + 2 × 3min at 5km race pace (90sec recovery) – w/down
Day 3	40min easy	40min easy	30min easy	w/up – 2 sets of 6 × 2min at 3km to 5km race pace (60sec jog and 3 min jog between sets) w/down	40min easy	40min easy	
Day 4	w/up – 5 × 10min at half-marathon pace (2min jog)	w/up – 30min at half-marathon pace + 20sec per mile; 10min at half-marathon pace; 6min at 10km pace	w/up – 25min at half-marathon pace + 15sec per mile	40min easy	w/up – 2 × 7 min at 10 mile race pace (90 sec jog) + 5 × 3 min at 3km race pace (90sec jog) w/down	w/up – 12min at half-marathon pace (90sec jog) – 4 × 4min at 5km race pace (90sec jog) – w/down	1 mile easy – 25min at half-marathon pace + 10 to 15sec per mile – 1 mile easy
Day 5							
Day 6	16 miles steady	17 miles steady		15 miles progressive e.g. 9 miles at half-marathon pace + 40sec per mile, last 5 miles at approx half-marathon pace + 20/30sec per mile	1 mile easy – 7 miles at half-marathon pace + 40sec per mile/5 miles at half-marathon pace + 10–15sec per mile	1 mile easy – 9 miles at half-marathon pace + 20/25sec per mile	
Day 7			10km or 10 mile race				Half-marathon race
Total Miles	43	43	31	36	42	35	29

responsibility. The following rules of thumb for the conversions are indicative:

- Five times your 10km PB minus 10 minutes equals your marathon potential. This can actually be 'beaten' by a couple of minutes by runners who adapt well to the longer distance.

- Double the race distance and add about 15–20 seconds per mile for race performance (closer to 20–25 seconds for slower runners).
- Marathon time should be between 106 and 107 per cent of your half-marathon time. The author prefers this to the more simplistic way of doubling your half-mara-

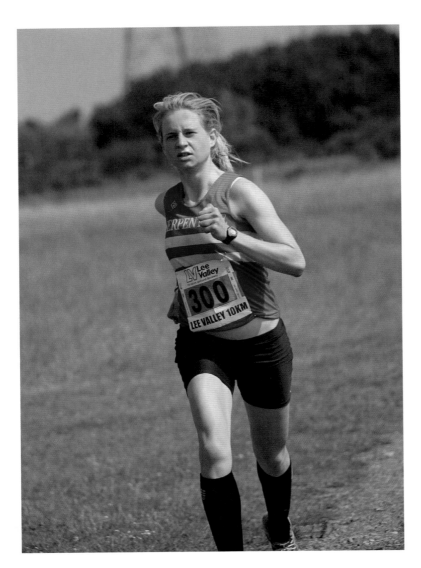

This 10km race was used as part of a half-marathon build-up.

22 miles into a marathon and some handle the relentless pace more evenly.

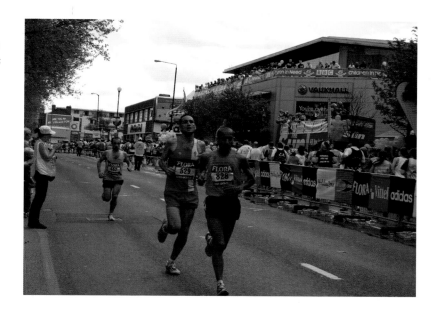

thon time and adding a certain number of minutes, because physiologically the percentage option can be more universally applied, whereas adding 4 minutes to a 67 minutes half-marathon PB is very different from adding it to a 1 hour 45 minute half-marathon time.

The key caveats for the above are:

- It is assumed that the runner has trained as specifically and thoroughly for the marathon as for 10km and in many cases this does not happen – most specifically in terms of just getting the mileage and long runs done on a consistent basis.
- The shorter-distance PBs are set on a similar course and terrain, and in similar weather conditions to what the marathon will offer, and that in overall fitness terms the runner facing the marathon starting pistol is physiologically the same beast who has done the 10km and half-marathons.

- Critically, that the pace in the marathon is done realistically and evenly. That leads into the next point.

During the Race

One thing we can all share, whether our marathon target is 2.10 or 3.59, is that it's a long time for a continuous sporting activity to be done, and that in the later stages it's going to hurt if we are running to our limit. So how do we deal with it? Former Australian marathon legend and the first World Champion in 1983, Rob de Castella, who pursued a career at director level in the Australian Institute of Sport, is always very shrewd on analysing the marathon. He described how at elite level dealing with the pain is in some ways just another factor for the mind to address, as is, for example, the weather, the crowds and any hills. However, at a more average running level the pain becomes the only issue dominating mind and body as we

75

enter the final miles. If we think about how elites analyse their marathon races compared to mid-packers it's a good insight – the latter will tend to focus far more on the final painful struggle, while the elites will look at the run more holistically.

There are perhaps some simple tricks ('strategies' in coaching parlance) that may help with this. Try not to start the race with your dominant mental focus being about a gradual approach of pain and struggle. Think about the race in stages, broken down into, for example, when you will take on drinks; when you may use a gel or two; how the course changes, both in the terrain/gradient (if applicable); and the surrounding environment and crowd support.

There is a physical and planning link to what your mind will have to tolerate in the later stages. If you misjudge the early pace and head off two quickly then the 'hitting the wall' scenario is inevitable. If you get to a level of serious discomfort at, say, 17 or 18 miles – not uncommon – then however positive you are, you just cannot escape that 8 or 9 miles in a state of suffering is a long, long way, and about an hour or more on the road. But if you do everything sensibly, the extreme level of discomfort may not hit you until about mile 24 – that is in line with the combination of maximum distance and pace that your training is likely to have covered, so something like 90 per cent of the total package. It is much more achievable for your mind to really push your body beyond what it has prepared for when it is 'just' another 10 per cent, or, in time on the road terms, maybe 15 minutes or so. It is easier to compare this to the last two miles of a training route and the relatively short stretch of road or country this will cover, than to visualize an 8- or 9-mile training route and convince your mind that it's just one last surge.

Preparing for Warm Weather Marathons

It is unlikely that international conferences about global warming focus unduly on how annoying climate changes can be for marathon runners chasing PBs. However, one aspect that has become a recurring feature in many spring and autumn marathons in Europe and the USA has been an unpredictability in the temperatures on race day. In recent years, major races such as London, Paris, Rotterdam, Boston, Chicago and Berlin have all experienced race-day weather that would be described as very warm or, exceptionally, hot. All of these races use the dates they do partly because generally they expect to get suitable long-distance running weather. This suits the races both athletically, as super-fast times at the sharp end are good for media coverage, and more generally because it means that the demands on medical and paramedical staff are likely to be far less onerous than if there are 35,000 runners enduring severe dehydration and heat stroke.

Very simply, hot temperatures impact adversely on endurance performance. Blood will be channelled more towards the skin surface to assist in keeping it cool, so less blood and therefore less oxygen are directed to the working muscles, with the result that aerobically the runner is in a less advantageous position. Because the body adapts to different challenges over time, there is a degree to which runners can prepare for warm weather marathons. This will not mean you will be likely to smash your marathon PB in temperatures of 25°C, but it might mean that, subject to sensible pacing and hydration, you may be within 1 or 2 minutes of your best time, rather than have a major collapse in performance.

For autumn marathons we are looking mainly at races between mid-September through to late October. One relevant factor is that a standard marathon preparation for such races will have included all the key long runs and hard training sessions over the summer months, so, one way or another, the athlete will have probably done some warm weather training practice even without any particular plan to do so.

For spring marathons the position is usually different. If you face an unseasonably warm day in mid-April, you may be given the awkward challenge of doing your hardest endurance run for many months in temperatures not faced for maybe six or seven months. Indeed, if it has been a particularly hard winter and you have done a two- or three-week taper reducing the longer runs, you may have not done any long runs for many weeks in a temperature above perhaps 10°C, in which case even 18–19°C is going to feel very uncomfortable in

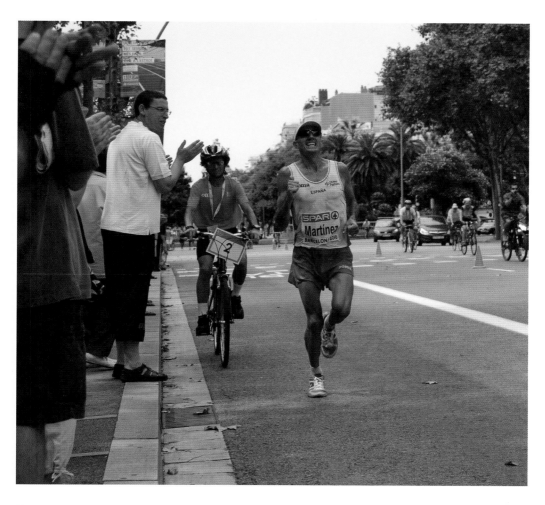

Hot weather marathons drain and dehydrate even the elite.

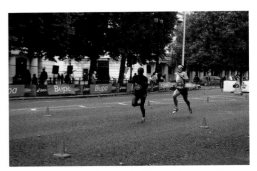

An evenly paced 10km or half-marathon can leave some capacity for a strong push to the finish line.

the later stages. (Of course, the usual scenario is that marathons start at about 9 o'clock in the morning so the hotter conditions are at least confined to the later stages.) Physically that is very tough and mentally it is not the most motivating scenario.

We will leave aside the options of travelling overseas to hot weather during the British winter or using a heat chamber at either a sports performance centre or a university, although both options are available. More practically, and free of cost or travel time, there is the simple but effective option of doing some of your longest runs and some of your harder threshold or marathon pace sessions in more clothing than feels totally comfortable. We are not talking thick fleeces and multiple layers of padded tracksuit pants – that would just cramp your movement capacity to run at the required pace and incur a level of heat exhaustion that would be counter-productive. But think about adding a thick cotton T-shirt, or even a light sweatshirt, plus a pair of tracksters to your normal gear for these sessions. Depending on what you are used to wearing and what sort of sweat rate you normally have, if you do maybe a handful of runs in your build-up with this extra clothing, that should bring some level of accli-

matization to your marathon day if it turns out to be warm.

Don't Forget About 10km

One of the requirements for runners who have strong marathon times relative to their 5km to 10km/10-mile performances must logically be that they need to improve their 5km/10km pace to set themselves up for further progress at the marathon. Otherwise, physiologically, you run out of spare capacity, because marathon pace becomes too close to 10km or 10-mile pace. This lends itself well to either having a spell, maybe one or two years, when you do just one marathon per year and thus spend most of the year not in specific marathon training. Or alternatively if you do two marathons a year, at approximately six-month intervals, you ensure that the marathon specifics and taper are contained within about twelve weeks each, which, even after recovery post-marathons and transition back to training, still leaves maybe five months per year where the focus is more on 5km/10km improvements.

Do not underestimate the challenge of a 10km race run at full effort. Spanish star Chema Martinez, European 10,000m champion in 2002 and frequently the best non-African in global championships, said 'That dread and anguish before a 10km never leaves me and is even worse than before a marathon.' You probably shouldn't be quite so anguished on the start line, but be prepared for the last 2–3km to be pretty painful as you try to maintain target pace. Although there are large numbers of 10km races available year round, their ubiquity does not make them any easier. Try to be selective in your 10km race choices and space them so that each one can be a test of how a new phase of training has been absorbed. Be realistic about how frequently you can trim your 10km PB, particularly if you run a best time on a dead flat course in ideal conditions, as you may not encounter this perfect scenario too frequently.

As shown earlier, the aerobic versus anaerobic split of energy requirements is very similar in both events, with barely 1 or 2 per cent provided by anaerobic glycolysis. Neither event should exhaust your glycogen supplies the way that marathons do and both distances fall within the standard definitions of 'long distance'. There is no need to provide a further set of training schedules that would have so much content in common with what has been presented already, so instead here are some general guidelines on what sort of adaptations to consider to the half-marathon schedules to make them more specific for improvements at 10km:

- Long runs can be capped at about 12 miles (or about 1 hour 45 minutes/1hour 50 minutes maximum) at this level and once you can manage these comfortably look to increase the pace in at least part of these runs.
- There is no need to assume that you need lower mileage for a 10km than for a half-

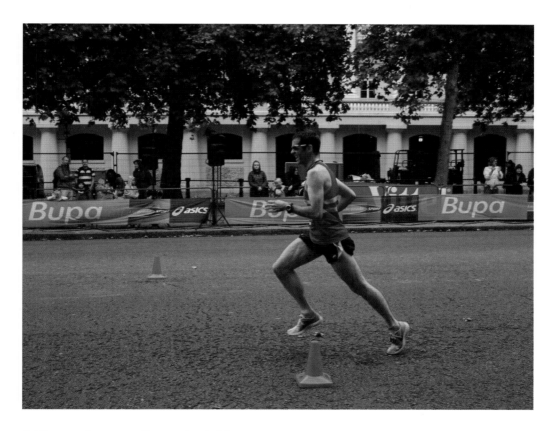

A 10km race forms part of a marathon build-up.

marathon. In terms of a 'get you round' option that may well be the case, but for the sort of improvements that rely on a challenging and progressive combination of steady state running, threshold sessions, hills and intervals and repetitions at close to your velocity at VO_2 max, the volumes are very similar.

- If anything, add an increased focus on running intervals at your notional 1,500m race pace instead of, or in addition to, sessions that focus on longer reps. You will not be doing these sort of sessions day in, day out, indeed far from it, but as a few of

examples of how you might plan a specific 10km session, consider these examples:

- **Session 1** 3 × 2km at 10km pace (2min recovery) + 3 × 1km at 5km pace (2min recovery) + 2 × 300m at 1,500 pace (1min recovery).
- **Session 2** 3km at 10-mile race pace/ slightly slower than threshold (2min recovery) + 1,600m/1 mile at 10km pace (90sec recovery) + 3 × 800m at 3km pace (90sec recovery) + 4 × 200m at 1,500m pace (30sec recovery).
- **Session 3** Three sets of (2km at threshold (90sec recovery) − 1,200m at 5km pace (2min recovery) − 300m at 1,500m pace (90sec recovery)).

The emphasis in these sessions, which are tough but definitely manageable if you get the pacing right, is more about running at very close to your vVO_2 max when you have already become fatigued after the first 6–7km of a 10km race, and indeed to run slightly quicker than this pace at the end of the session. There is nothing wrong in using sessions such as these as part of a marathon or half-marathon plan, but they would be more about underpinning the event-specific training, whereas for a 10km runner these sessions would be very specific for racing that distance. A subtle difference, but one worth considering as your training evolves.

CHAPTER 5

AEROBIC CROSS-TRAINING

Overview

This chapter is separated from that on strength and conditioning (Chapter 8) because its content is related to activities that can in some way replace or replicate the benefits of running training, whilst the strength and conditioning elements are aspects that support and supplement the running.

With the main element of your running being your cardiovascular efficiency, it is logical that any activity that can challenge you in a similar way to running is of some use. The world of cross-training and how it crosses over with running has changed considerably in the last twenty or thirty years, with these various factors all contributing:

- The growth of the triathlon, with the sporting loyalties of many runners split between cycling and swimming as a matter of course, means that their running performance will always have some short- or longer-term cross-training programme supporting it.
- The growth of the gym culture, so that many new runners enter the sport from a medley of cross-training modules via their gym, particularly steppers, spin bikes and elliptical trainers. With no background in a 'traditional' running environment they have evolved their running as part of a broader aerobic programme.
- Arguably there is a less hardy approach to running 'in all weathers' so that, linked to the growth in gym membership, runners may more readily trade running for a cross-training session when the weather outside is particularly bad. In the depths of winter this may be great common-sense and an injury-avoidance technique that some hardened harriers might consider.
- There is greater precision and empathy in the sports medical world so that whereas in bygone years the advice to an injured runner might be to stop running and do a suitable remedial set of conditioning drills, nowadays there will be a more specific and runner-friendly approach to what aerobic training can be carried out whilst the running is on the back-burner.
- The increasing use of the Internet and social media has made more recreational runners aware of how elite endurance athletes may incorporate cross-training into their running build-up, either as a regular integral element, or more usually as a way of rehabbing an injury without compromising aerobic fitness.

As with all aspects of training, you will need to work out a balance of what suits your own particular circumstances and level of commitment. Don't lose sight of the importance of event- and sport-specificity. If cross-training was absolutely transferable across sports then in theory a Tour de France cyclist should be able to crack out a 2.15 marathon and the mighty East African half-marathon elite should be able to hop on a bike and demolish the cycling world in a 1-hour road race. Anyone who saw how hard the USA cycling legend Lance Armstrong had to work just to sneak under 3 hours in a marathon will see the point.

Conversely, one of the GB marathoners selected for the Olympic Marathon in late August 2004 spent about ten weeks in the middle of what would have been the specific build-up unable to run because of injury. In this ten-week spell the athlete largely mirrored what would have been the duration, heart rate and intensity of their running training by using an elliptical cross-trainer and spin bike. The injury gradually cleared in time to do a short spell of key running sessions and the athlete had a fine result in Athens.

A case of what might have been? Maybe in part, but also a reflection that the aerobic quality of the non-running training was thoroughly planned with the Athens goal in mind and the runner was clearly highly motivated to train hard towards the Olympic goal. Plus there would have been a large amount of running 'carry forward' from the training that the athlete had done in preparation for the London Marathon in April 2004, which had secured the Olympic selection.

This chapter will not address in detail how cross-training can be used to keep fit while too injured to run, as that will vary case by case with the nature of the injury and in light of individual medical advice. Rather, it looks more generally at how the various options may work for you. The overarching premise should be that your training for running should optimally be running. When for whatever reason you adapt aerobic cross-training, you should aim to keep the two or three key sessions each week as running to maximize the specificity of the training stimulus and the cross-training should mainly be used as additional basic, steady state work.

Some scientific research on this subject has looked at fit, well-trained runners in the 18–19-minute range for 5km and had one group add three runs to their weekly training, whilst the second group added the same duration in three cycling sessions. The improvements in 5km results after two months were very similar in both groups, which endorses the benefits of aerobic cross-training. However, it's worth emphasizing that in this research both groups did their more intense sessions as running throughout the period.

Cycling

Typically, 1 mile of cycling at a given intensity or heart rate is 'worth' about one quarter of a mile of comparable running effort in aerobic benefit. This means that to match the training effect of a 1-hour run, very roughly you may need to cycle between 90 minutes and 2 hours, depending on your running level versus your cycling proficiency. This is a combination of the fact that cycling uses less of your total muscle groups than running does and also any downhill freewheeling on the bike would require less effort than running at an even pace down the same descent. This 'equation' is one reason why a typical triathlon programme will have much more time spent on the bike than on running.

Runners doing hard sessions on a bike, even a stationary bike, will invariably find that at the higher levels of effort, including absolute maximum, they will have heart rates about 5–7 beats per minute lower than when running at the same perceived effort. This is partly because of the fewer muscle groups engaged and also because whereas a trained competitive cyclist will have developed powerful leg muscles to drive the bike at maximum cardiovascular effort, a 'mere' runner's legs will not be as specifically prepared to divert so much energy through the upper legs.

Elliptical Cross-Trainer

This is perhaps the closest replication to running with the great advantage of having no impact. The distribution of effort across the body's main muscle groups is very close to that of running. Using your preferred combination of heart rate or perceived effort you can carry out any number of training sessions, from an easy pace through to aerobic power work, at about your 3–5km notional race-pace effort. It is harder to go at a higher effort than this as runners' biomechanics and the structure of the machine seems to prevent the rapidity of movement needed to get the heart rate towards its absolute maximum. Perhaps because there is no impact, when doing interval or repetition sessions you may find that the recovery needed between reps is slightly less than when doing comparable running sessions.

As with all cross-training done indoors, be aware that the lack of any air resistance, often coupled with a higher air temperature than outdoors, will lead to a far higher loss of sweat than doing the same session outdoors. About 1ltr of fluid and electrolyte replacement per hour should be taken on board, ideally during the session, and topped up promptly after finishing, when you will probably continue to sweat at this increased rate for some minutes.

Aquajogging/Water Running

The dual title for this activity is intended to show that it has a serious and useful benefit for improving performance and need not simply be a base-level aerobic activity. Running in water provides a non-impact workout that exercises the same muscles as if you were running on land. It is tiring and, unlike normal running, it is much easier to lose your balance in the water. Keep in mind that you will get tired faster doing this than normal running because each stride is against the resistance of water.

Deep-water running takes place in a deep pool without your feet touching the bottom, floating in place with the help of a flotation belt. Because the feet do not touch the ground, deep-water running is completely non-impact, making it perfect for those with vulnerable knees. For a proper deep-water exercise, lean slightly forwards in the water, avoiding a straight up-and-down posture that won't give the workout its full impact as it will bring in assisted 'bobbing' movement due to the belt's buoyancy effect. Also avoid the lower leg (that is, below the knee) coming forwards past the knee – a movement that may occur in the water, but is not how you would run on land.

Shallow-water running involves a regular pool, with the feet actually touching the bottom. Because of this, it is slightly higher impact than deep-water running, but is still much lower than traditional running. With feet making contact with a surface, the shallow-water option more closely resembles regular running. As such, it is helpful for increasing running speed and strength. The exercise is done in much the same way as in deep water, but because the feet are making contact to help propel you forwards it is often done somewhat more slowly. If using a heart-rate monitor, expect that for a given rate of effort your heart rate will be about 5–10 per cent slower than in 'normal' running.

The fairly obvious less appealing factors about water running are that the time required to do a session is much longer than doing a comparable running session. If you have access to a swimming pool at a work-based gym, this can help on the time-management side. Mentally, of course, the four walls of a swimming pool tend to be less varied and stimulating than even a fairly humdrum running route, so you will need to form sort of mental distraction to make sessions less boring. Doing some sort of intervals or fartlek or at least varied efforts helps with this, as well as heightening the aerobic training stimulus by ensuring that not every minute is exactly the same as the preceding and succeeding minute. There are also some organized coached groups doing structured water-running sessions, although these are relatively few at the current time.

Swimming

The big advantage of swimming is that there is no impact, so the risk of running injuries is negligible. The downside is that the transferability of swimming fitness to endurance running is generally less than that provided by the other cross-training options. The cardiovascular element is of course excellent and, generally, can be as hard as you wish to make it provided you are able to swim continuously, so as a maintenance option that is fine. But of course the muscle groups used in swimming, and the way they are used, vary significantly from those used in running.

Another possible limitation is that to provide a structured aerobic session, as opposed to just continued lengths at a steady state, one does need a certain level of technical proficiency to be able to swim at a relaxed, slow effort when, for example, a recovery training session is planned, or if an interval session is planned with varying paces. As evidence for the importance of technical competence, the British Triathlon Federation's elite talent programmes will focus on youngsters with a swimming and running background where the skill can be taught young, and to a high level, whereas cycling can be moulded on later. Conversely, in his coaching manual/autobiography, triathlon legend Scott Tinsley

describes seeing a lean, fit young man spluttering through swimming 25m lengths at more than 40 seconds each and exclaiming 'What the hell? I'm a 2.27 marathoner!'

For those runners who do have a good level of swimming technique, one advantage is that they can carry out hard, structured training, which, although it may be fatiguing in terms of aerobic challenge, does not produce that muscular wear and tear in the legs that comparably tough road or track running sessions will cause.

Rowing/Indoor Rower/ Canoe Ergo

The widespread availability of indoor rowers, usually the Concept 2 machines, linked perhaps to the continued international success and high profile of British rowing, has kept rowing in the forefront of cross-training. Indeed, indoor rowing now exists as a sport in its own right with various competitions available.

The indoor rowing motion is technically quite easy to master to a level of competency that makes it suitable for use as a cardiovascular element of running training. The simplicity of the movement, provided you are doing it with the lower back and hamstrings correctly positioned and used, and the fact that the machines are invariably set up with computers to indicate speed and distance, along with sensors monitoring heart rate, means that any sort of interval or repetition session can be done on a rowing machine in addition to continuous steady-state training.

Less widespread are the canoeing world's equivalent of the indoor rower, where a simulated canoe paddle is used as the main tool of resistance with the athlete sitting on a machine that otherwise closely resembles a Concept 2. The same sort of training points are applicable here, with the added factor that the paddling movement is slightly more technically precise than ploughing ahead on the rower. Currently these items are about triple the cost of indoor rowers, hence they are less widely available but they serve a useful aerobic purpose.

Rowing and canoeing place great emphasis on upper body strength and endurance, far more than endurance running does, and the body shape of high-level athletes in these sports shows this clearly. So the transferability of the training benefit is not as high as that provided by cycling or the elliptical cross-trainer. The London Marathon performances of the likes of Stephen Redgrave and James Cracknell show the point clearly. Chapter 6 describes a case history of how paddle-sport training helped a runner to improve his performances.

KEY POINTS

- Assess which cross-training options seem to have most transferrable benefit for running.
- Bloody mindedness is an asset for cross-training.
- Seek cross-training options that are feasible within your other commitments and accept that most are less time-efficient than running.
- Varying the pace and effort of cross-training has a major effect on reducing the boredom factor.

CHAPTER 6

VETERANS' RUNNING

The Background

Go to almost any long-distance road race outside national elite competition and the first thing you may notice is the large number of runners who are slightly past their first flush of youth. In fact, it may be difficult to pick out any runners in their early or mid-twenties, their physical prime. The typical sports participation pathway that modern British people – and much of the Western world – follow is that whatever level of sports they do until age fourteen to sixteen at school, they gradually do less and less as they get older. It is a varied combination of computer games and educational, social and career pressures

that collectively produces a very inactive adult population.

Fortunately for the world of distance running there is a significant minority of people who buck this trend and make some lifestyle changes in, typically, their thirties and forties. They are looking to regain some level of fitness and for many jogging or running fits the bill. Compared to most other sports, running is, at its most basic level, simple to do, cheap and easy to start (you can't go sailing or horse riding just by putting on some trainers and starting the activity as soon as you have closed the front door behind you). It is also often simple to make noticeable improvements as a novice.

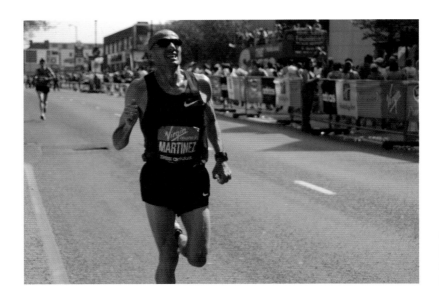

An exceptional forty-year-old still competing at elite level.

Although many veterans or masters competitions include a thirty-five to thirty-nine age group, this chapter will consider veteran running to start at forty. Long-distance runners are very much at the height of their endurance prowess at age thirty-five, which they can hold for a further two or three years, so we really should see age forty as when some of the 'vets only' factors start to come into play.

Depending on a whole host of factors, these new runners often become hooked and are as much a part of the running community as the high performers at county and regional level. Indeed, in some cases they actually become the leading county and regional runners if they have been blessed with good genes and follow a high-performance training plan for some years. The fastest world performances in the various age categories over forty are in their way as mind-blowing as the world records in the standard senior ranks. Indeed, the marks by forty year olds are mighty impressive within the open categories, for example a sub-2.09 male marathon and a 2.26 woman's marathon.

So in many ways the best practice guidelines for senior runners can be and are applicable to veteran runners. However, there are various factors that runners over forty need to consider, which younger runners may be able to put on the back burner for some years.

Long May You Run

In researching his book on veteran runners, Bruce Tulloh's survey of over 200 forty-pluses found 'as many different patterns as there are individuals', which chimes neatly with this author's view that 'each athlete is an experiment of one'. We've all seen those questionnaires asking why we run, with reasons from 'Wanting to compete for Great Britain' to 'Being able to eat plenty of cake without turning into Michelin Man' and covering factors such as health and fitness; desire to test one's limits; bringing structure and contrast to a busy but often sedentary lifestyle; and social networks.

Most of these factors will apply to most runners, but the relative priority will vary immensely. The Olympic runner won't be running 120 miles a week to make more friends or ensure her jeans fit well, but she will be aware that these are positive results from her running life. The man trying to beat 90 minutes for a half-marathon won't relocate to an Ethiopian hillside to achieve this, but he might moderate his Saturday night beer and curry intake. Experienced runners who face the inevitable fact that as they get past their late thirties and particularly into their mid-to-late forties their race times will be heading south, may change their running goals and priorities, perhaps in ways they would not have expected in earlier years.

As a couple of contrasting examples of outliers, Abel Anton, who followed a uniquely Spanish career path from abattoir assistant to world-class distance runner, won his second World Championship marathon, in Seville, in front of his compatriots, aged thirty-seven, in 1999, having run a PB of 2.07 earlier that year to win the Flora London Marathon. Two years later he was retired from elite athletics. Hypothetically, if he had stayed as a full-time runner he would have been running maybe 2.11 or 2.12 – fantastic stuff of course, but that 2 per cent loss in performance would probably have made the athletics much less financially viable and we could guess that the unique emotional highs of crossing the line to become World Champion would not be matched. But he never sought further employment at the abattoir.

At the same age as Anton was winding down, British maestro Keith Anderson was just ramping up the high-performance gears. In his early thirties he led a sedentary lifestyle. He was a chef in the Lake District, overweight and smoking twenty-five cigarettes a day. He followed a belated path to high-performance endurance, culminating in a 48.16 10-mile race (a UK record that will take some beating), and a 2.17 marathon aged forty-one, which secured him selection for the Commonwealth Games where he placed ninth. In his fifth decade he was living as a professional runner, pushing out the barriers with extended training trips to the high altitude of Kenya and funding the lifestyle with targeted road races in the UK and USA. We'll never know what he would have run if he had had this focus in his twenties or early thirties, or indeed if an earlier peak would have sapped his physical and mental capacity to hit such heights in his forties.

However, aside from the inspiring case histories, there are trends – look at the world age category records in the tables below. Once you've done with marvelling at how people of these ages can run so fast, you will notice that invariably these global marks are set by athletes in the first year or two of the relevant five-year age bands. Statistically inclined readers can also do the maths to monitor the rate of decline. By and large it is in the region of 2–4 seconds per mile per year.

The Best of the Best

In terms of what you as a forty-plus might achieve, if all or most of the following apply you might still have some latent PBs in the tank:

- Less than five years of any regular running.
- Less than two years of 'proper' structured and challenging running training.
- Carrying a few extra kilos of weight.
- Never really focused on what you might achieve as a runner beyond general aerobic fitness.
- Poor nutritional and alcohol habits.
- Never spent quality time on any non-running training elements relating to strength/strength endurance; flexibility; technique and running form.

The Best of the Best

Men's Marathon Age Group	Mark	Name	Country	Age
M 40	2:08:46	Andrés Espinosa	MEX	
M 45	2:15:51	Kjell-Erik Ståhl	SWE	45
M 50	2:19:29	Titus Mamabolo	RSA	
M 55	2:25:56	Piet van Alphen	NED	55
M 60	2:36:30	Yoshihisa Hosaka	JPN	60
M 65	2:41:57	Derek Turnbull	NZL	65
M 70	2:54:48	Ed Whitlock	CAN	73

Men's 10,000 Track Age Group	Mark	Name	Country	Age
M 40	28:30:88	Martii Vainio	FIN	40
M 45	30:02:56	Antonio Villaneuva	MEX	45
M 50	30:55:16	Peter de Vocht	BEL	50
M 55	32:27:7	Michael F. Hager	GBR	55
M 60	34:14:88	Luciano Acquarone	ITA	60
M 65	34:42:2	Derek Turnbull	NZL	65
M 70	38:04:13	Ed Whitlock	CAN	70
M 75	39:25:16	Ed Whitlock	CAN	75

Women's 10,000 Track Age Group	Mark	Name	Country	Age
W 40	31:40:97	Alla Zhilyaeva	RUS	40
W 45	32:34:06	Evy Palm	SWE	46
W 50	35:41:90	Gitte Karlshöj	DEN	50
W 55	37:09:4	Sandra Branney	GBR	55
W 60	39:04:23	Bernadine Portenski	NZL	60
W 65	42:07:1	Theresia Baird	AUS	65
W 70	47:22:51	Melitta Czerwenka-Nagel	GER	70
W 70	50:00:93	Melitta Czerwenka-Nagel	GER	70

Women's Marathon Age Group	Mark	Name	Country	Age
W 40	2:26:51	Priccilla Welch	GBR	42
W 45	2:29:00	Tatyana Pozdnyakova	UKR	46
W 50	2:48:47	Edeltraud Pohl	FRG	52
W55	2:52:14	Rae Baymiller	USA	
W 60	3:14:50	Barbara Miller	USA	
W 65	3:28:10	Lieselotte Schultz	FRG	
W 70	3:46:18	Ginette Bedard	USA	72
W 75	4:10:07	Betty Jean McHugh	CAN	

Clearly we can't quantify the performance gains related to any of the above, but the author suggests that they are listed in order of relative significance. To illustrate this, one can find international marathoners with rather sketchy credentials on the two final factors, but you will be unlikely to unearth a runner of that level who hasn't ticked the first two boxes.

Age Grading – Measuring Up

Most veteran readers will be aware of the age grading tables, a simple mathematical calculation that uses the world age best for each single age in each event, so that every performance can be shown as a percentage of the world's best. So a man of forty-six doing a 92-minute half-marathon can compare his result to, for example, a woman of forty-one doing 97 minutes in the same race. It is not unusual for the top age-graded performance at an event to be by someone who does not feature at the very front of the race. For runners who have reached an age and stage where their absolute times are slowing down, maintaining or improving their age-graded rating can be a highly motivating factor for some. Generally, those who came to the sport later in life seem to be more focused on this benchmarking of performance, whereas the traditional Harrier types who have come through the ranks as youngsters tend to be less driven by the stats – even though they may be running fairly swiftly.

Runners might also consider the vets-only championships at County, Area and National levels. The marathon and half-marathon championships are invariably held within existing events, which vary annually. Results are sorted on a five-yearly category basis, although everyone races together at these longer events (unlike the 5km and 10km

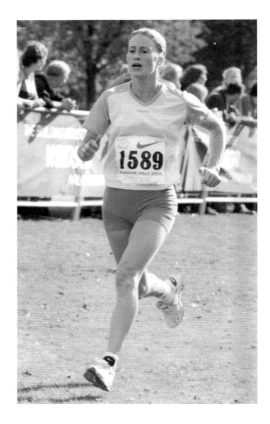

Aged forty, this runner broke 3 hours in 2011 in her second marathon.

races). Although the standard at the front is very high, the very existence of these events can provide a useful focus for planning and motivation. The result, enabling the runner to achieve a specific position in a regional or national event, seems possibly a more solid outcome than just another time in another open event. Runners need to be affiliated to the relevant Governing Body (England Athletics or Home Country equivalent) to be eligible for these events and the results down the field are probably less daunting than many might guess.

Veteran Medical Factors

Some veteran 'focus areas' have been high-lighted by physical therapist Gerard Hart-mann, who has great medical credentials in endurance sport. As a key physiother-apy back-up provider to the likes of Paula Radcliffe, World Champion Sonia O'Sullivan and Olympic 1,500 Champion Noah Ngeny of Kenya, amongst many other big hitters, he is considered in the endurance running world to have 'magic hands' because of the precision of his diagnoses and treatments. His most nota-ble veteran link was with Irish legend Eamonn Coghlan, who ran a 3.58 mile aged forty-one, which is a staggering run at that age.

He precedes the specifics by suggesting that 'stress is the most silent killer. Everyone has a different tolerance to stress and it is very much individually registered'. This is not the forum to look in detail at the huge diversity of people's lifestyles, but as a general practi-cal point for runners he says 'Many athletes squeeze their training into hectic workdays – I question the wisdom of this.' Of course, how you balance this if your pursuit of endurance prowess is unavoidably and inextricably bound up with factors like a full-time job, parenting of young children, travelling to and from work, and some sort of family and social network where not everyone builds their plans around your PB-hunting, is where each individual has to sort out what works best.

He does, however, focus on veteran runners maintaining a lower bodyweight, usually linked to a lower percentage of body fat for all the usual reasons related to performance, recov-ery, injury prevention and – linked to an ample intake of anti-oxidants – a healthy immune system. In addition:

- Muscle strength and muscle mass fall between about 30–50 per cent between the ages of thirty and seventy. The strength

and conditioning elements covered in Chapter 8 are therefore highly relevant to veterans – if anything, they are even more fundamental because as the joints in the knees, hips and ankles weaken through age, they are ever more vulnerable to injury if the major and core muscle groups are not taking their optimum share of the impact of running.

- Flexibility decreases as the body's collagen and elasticin content change in composi-tion. Hartmann unequivocally suggests 'at least ten minutes per day' of stretching.
- The above is linked to his recommenda-tion to keep some faster-paced running as a regular training element and the prepa-ration for and execution of this pace will involve dynamic stretching to maintain or at least constrain the decreasing range of movement that nature is causing.
- Also linked to flexibility and elasticity are running drills that break down the running movement into key elements and look at maximizing the quality of these. These include:

- fast feet, moving as if you are stepping on hot coals, so minimizing ground contact;
- high knees, done as a walk-through with one foot on the ground at all times, bring-ing the knee up through to waist level, keeping the trunk held high and erect;
- once the high-knees drill is done effi-ciently, an exaggerated arm action should be brought in, so that as the thigh is raised the opposite hand is brought up to the forehead, ensuring it does not cross the body.

Typically, do each drill for about 10 seconds, about three times – this duration is about the time to get into and repeat the movement to whatever is your best level, and stopping before fatigue creeps in and compromises the quality of movement and also probably your concentration.

Joint Problems

This section is about osteoarthritis, because for ageing runners it is perhaps the most frequent injury problem that is veteran-specific. We've all had the naysayers telling us how 'all that wear and tear on the legs' must be damaging in the long term, and in particular the threat of osteoarthritis.

Clearly in a degenerative condition that affects a significant number of people in middle and older age, there are going to be numerous runners who also suffer from it – that is just simple statistics and probability. Fortunately there is some robust research and maybe the most informative is the data used by Arthritis Research and Therapy obtained from the Fifty Plus Runners Association in the USA. Over a fourteen-year timescale it compared runners as they progressed through their fifties and sixties, with a control group of non-runners. The runners averaged 26 miles per week training, regular but not truly high mileage as such. The runners experienced 'about 25 per cent less musculo-skeletal pain than the non-runners'. It is notable that this is a perception by the runners that is not actually a medical diagnosis, but for practical purposes it is sensible to know how we will feel as we continue running in our later years. Arthritis Research UK has stated directly: 'The stronger the muscles and tissues around your joints, the better they will be able to support and protect those joints. If you don't exercise, your muscles become smaller and weaker.'

The caveat to this is when a runner has had an injury around a joint and the nature of the healing process, combined with a return to running that has maybe continued to 'stretch the envelope' more than is ideal and is well in excess of those 26 miles per week mentioned above, has left a structural weakness. Over time, this does indeed leave the area vulnerable to osteoarthritis. Research indicates that in 75 per cent of sports people with the disease, it is on a site where there has been a previous injury to the affected joint that has adversely affected the quantity or strength of the cartilage; in the large majority of runners, this will be the knee.

Supplements for Osteoarthritis

Collagen hydrolysate supplements are rich in amino-acids, which have a key role in synthesizing collagen, a major component of joint cartilage. So the simple theory is that rebuilding and/or strengthening existing cartilage can ease the symptoms of arthritis. Arthritis Research UK's latest position on this is that relevant trials 'are scarce and yielded mixed results'. It rates its effectiveness as two out of five. So it's not a miracle cure for all and the tests are not runner-specific. However, if you are one of those runners for whom the 'two out of five' score has a practical benefit that enables you to run with less discomfort, it may be worth checking out.

Chondroitin sulphate exists naturally in your body and is thought to give elasticity to cartilage and to slow its breakdown. In supplement form it is often taken alongside glucosamine to relieve the symptoms of osteoarthritis. There is no proof that it reverses cartilage loss, but some studies suggest it helps to stop joint degeneration. Chondroitin is a slow-acting supplement, so do not expect to see any improvement for at least two months. It doesn't help everyone – if you have severe cartilage loss you probably won't get any benefit. There do not appear to be any serious side-effects, but minor ones include occasional nausea and indigestion. It could increase your chances of bleeding if you are taking any blood-thinning drugs. The long-term effects of taking chondroitin are not known.

Depending on the product and the level of bulk buying you commit to, supplements based on the compounds above typically cost about £20–25 for a month's supply.

Each runner should bear in mind that the rate at which the problem may worsen will vary between individuals. But a more universal factor is that on each long run the shock-absorption traits of the joints are weakened in the latter miles, which may lead some affected runners to bid farewell to marathon training and running, and to focus their efforts towards 10km and maybe half-marathons, with a view to 'running longevity' that continued marathons may jeopardize. Bear in mind that the above-mentioned survey average of 26 miles per week would probably not have included many very long runs – let's use 15 miles as a watershed for this purpose, as the sort of distance where marathon-specificity comes into play.

Recovery and Training Structures

One trend that very few ageing runners will be able to ignore is that the time needed to recover between hard sessions, and indeed between any training sessions, becomes longer. We need to respect this and work out constructive ways to manage this without it affecting performance more than is necessary. Even runners in their mid-to-late thirties performing at the very highest level acknowledge that they have to revise some of their training habits from ten years earlier.

Certainly the practice of doing harder efforts on alternate days three times per week, which is difficult to sustain at any age, becomes very hard to manage successfully in the veterans age groups, particularly if there is a purposeful long run to be done at the weekend.

Tim Noakes' authoritative book, *The Lore of Running*, even goes so far as to advise veteran runners to look at a planned programme of alternate days of running and cross-training (cycling, in the examples he mentions), with a couple of case histories of how at a high level the performances at 10km seemed to thrive off this balance. One case was an ex-Olympic runner with a 28.30 PB who was nudging 32 minutes in his mid-forties. Great running, undoubtedly, but he needed to deal physically and mentally with a drop-off rate of some 35 seconds per mile over about fifteen years, which is within the typical range of decline mentioned earlier. The volume and duration of cycling mentioned was substantial, so this isn't a cop-out but an alternative means to strong performance. This is worth considering, though his recommendations did not cover:

- What sort of age these concessions to the ageing process should start, so someone aged thirty-nine and three-quarters running six days a week should not expect just to cut the mileage in half as soon as they hit forty.
- The balance of the harder sessions and recovery sessions between running and cross-training.
- How applicable this would be to half-marathon and marathon runners.

There are no hard and fast rules on the frequency of sessions but some of the following should be kept in mind:

- If you are not already doing so, look at training in terms of what you want to cover in a fourteen- or twenty-eight-day period, rather than a brief seven-day weekly cycle.

- Where lifestyle commitments allow, do not be bound to rituals on certain days of the week. It is often hard to find time and energy for very long runs on days within a Monday to Friday working pattern, but with the increasing options of family-friendly working life there may be flexibility. Also do not feel obliged to turn up at the club or group Tuesday reps session just because it's there and it's Tuesday. When planning your training it may be enlightening just to number the days 1 to 14 or 1 to 28, rather than feel constrained by what a given day usually entails. As an extreme case of how we can get stuck in our ways, the author was once asked by a runner if there was some biological or biorhythmic reason why the body could not train hard on a Friday, as all the training schedules she'd seen in magazines and websites always showed Friday as a rest day.

- Think about maybe four harder efforts per fourteen days, or five harder efforts per twenty-one days and accept that as you get older you will probably have to gradually increase the number of recovery/easy days in-between the harder efforts.

- However, do still push the harder efforts as much as you did when you were younger. The race distances are not shortened to reflect your added years, and 100 per cent effort is 100 per cent effort at any age, though the speed at which ground can be covered at 100 per cent effort may be reduced. That said, the graphic, though not empirically proven mantra, that 'a hard training session isn't hard enough unless you throw up' has only ever been related to the author by athletes on the young side of forty.

- Some of the advice in Chapter 5 about aerobic cross-training may become more relevant as you age. The balancing act between preparing specifically to do long-distance road races and protecting your joints from the repeated impact of long-distance road running will evolve over time. You cannot prepare thoroughly and exclusively by cross-training, but you may think about doing some of the steady-state training as non-running, interspersed between the harder efforts done on the run. You might also look to mix and match some of the longer runs, so that, for example, a 2¼-hour long session might comprise 90 minutes running then 45 minutes on a cross-training option, ideally done as closely as possible to the end of the run. The cardiovascular, aerobic and fat-burning effects will be very similar for a given level of intensity, but the exponential wear and tear on the joints of the final miles of a long training run would be avoided.

Integration of Cross-Training

Below are two typical simple schedules followed by a man of forty-five who was running the occasional 10km in 38–38.30. He had a PB of 33.00 set twenty years earlier when he had regularly run around 80–90 miles per week and was about 11lb (5kg) lighter. The obvious major difference is the running volume. The fact that after adhering to both schedules for some months the running performance was very similar is consistent with Noakes' comments.

The other more subtle difference is that the elliptical gives a slightly less intense challenge than running, so that repetitions that could be run at something between 1,500m or 3–5km pace tended to be more like 5–10km effort on the cross-trainer. So the intense sessions on the elliptical tend to go for slightly longer reps; slightly less recovery and slightly more total

Cross-Training Dominant

M	40min easy run inc 7 or 8 × 20sec strides
T	X-trainer – w/up then alternate weekly sessions of e.g. 10 × 3min at 5km effort, with 60sec 'jog' or 5 × 6min at 10km effort with 60sec 'jog'
W	50min easy run
T	55/60min easy steady run
F	X-trainer – around threshold effort, for example simulation of 'out and back' session of 25min at notional half-marathon effort followed by 20min at 10km to 10-mile race pace
S	rest
S	elliptical X-trainer – 2hr, first hour to 70min easy/comfortable, last 50/60min at notional marathon effort
Total aerobic volume	20 miles easy to steady running plus 3 harder X-training sessions

Running Dominant

M	55min easy X-trainer
T	Running – interval session alternating weeks of for example 6 or 7 × 4.5min c.5km pace with 2min jog recovery with 11 or 12 × 2min reps at c.3km pace with 60sec recovery
W	50min easy run
T	60min steady pace run
F	Harder running session – alternate weeks of w/up then 45/50min sustained running progressing from notional marathon pace to about 10-mile race pace, alternate with long reps at about 10-mile race pace e.g. 4 × 10 or 11min with 2min jog of 5 × 8 or 9min with 90sec jog
S	rest
S	1hr 45 to 1hr 50 run, easy start, last 30min at notional marathon effort
Total aerobic volume	47 miles running inc 2 harder sessions plus one easy X-training session

duration of reps than running sessions would entail. The occasional short rep session on the cross-trainer would be something like thirty-two to thirty-five reps of 35–40 seconds done at about 3km effort (by perceived rate of effort) on a 60-second cycle – thus giving a recovery of 20 or 25 seconds. It is slightly less gruelling on the cross-trainer, because if done as a running session the aim would be to pace it at very close to your speed at VO_2 max – or vVO_2 max, to represent 'velocity' – whereas on an elliptical it is hard to make the arm and leg movement quick enough to achieve this intensity. It may suit whirling dervishes though.

In another upbeat case history, the author has coached for some years a mid-forties runner with a keen interest in canoeing. During this period the athlete never ran more than four times a week, more usually three times. He combined this with, for most of the year, one or two structured and tough canoe sessions and one strength/strength-endurance session each week. During this period, between the ages of forty-three and forty-six and having already got three years of running training in the bank, his marathon time improved by 8 minutes and his half-marathon time by 4 minutes, at an age when it is usually hard for seasoned runners to prevent some slippage. This is also in the context that the muscular endurance in canoeing has different priorities compared to running – just look at elite canoeists' upper bodies to illustrate this. However, to show how, cardiovascularly, endurance coaches are singing from a similar hymn sheet in various sports, there was one bittersweet day when the athlete did a running session of 25 reps of 200m in the morning, then pitched up at the canoe club in the evening where the club session was 24 reps of 200m.

It is a simplistic summary of the above to suggest that our view of how veterans run is about whether we see the glass as half full or half empty. However, many of us will have some days when we think 'I'm only a few years past my very peak, I'm in great shape, motivated and experienced' and others when,

with morning soreness, maybe a slight rounding of the tummy or buttocks, and a set of 800m reps done at what used to be slower than our marathon pace, we feel that nature is having its way.

KEY POINTS

- Although every individual case may vary, there are inevitable trends of how increased age after the late thirties affects one's capacity for endurance performance.
- Strength and conditioning is at least as vital for masters runners as for younger ones.
- There is no need to reduce the intensity or volume of harder sessions for veteran runners, but the timescale for recovery from them is likely to increase.
- There is some persuasive evidence of how certain supplements can help to preserve joints' strength.
- Integrating regular cross-training may help to achieve a balance between keeping performance at a good level, reducing injury frequency and extending one's running longevity.

PART II

THE RUNNING BODY

CHAPTER 7

RUNNING MOVEMENT AND TECHNICAL ASPECTS

The Principles

When endurance coaching gurus are asked to put into a single sentence what they would seek to instil in any successful runner, they will invariably make reference to having sound technical running form. This is because in terms of efficiency of movement, or the biomechanical aspect of 'running efficiency', this will enable the runner to cover the distance quicker. It will also usually be linked to a lower incidence of injury.

That's the simple part. The more difficult part is analysing what comprises sound technique, then applying that to each individual runner, and then the runner spending the necessary time developing the best technique they can. Let's be realistic and accept that amongst the many reasons why people become involved in long-distance running, practising running drills is very rarely part of the attraction. The busier you are in your life, the more you will want to prioritize your training time on doing the running rather than doing the activities that support the running.

But reflect on what you are trying to achieve, both in the running and the supplementary training. If you isolate one tough training session in a five-month block of preparation – let's say six reps of 5 minutes at about 10km pace with a 60-second jog recovery – how much actual impact on performance does that one session have amidst what may be well over 100 running sessions? Not much, but it is hard work and will take an hour or so of your time, all told. What if you spent 1 hour broken down into four blocks of 15 minutes, during each of which you spent quality time developing your running technique along good biomechanical lines? Would the benefit be any more or less than the notional rep session?

We don't know exactly, but one thing we can identify from watching elite endurance runners is that almost without exception they move efficiently. How they have developed this ease and grace of movement will vary immensely, and indeed there will be an element of genetic luck in their body type and their musculoskeletal structures. There will be athletes who as children were well taught in running movement years before they ever had a focus on distance running. Others may have had some specialism in different sports involving running, been coached within that particular sport and later transferred this skill into distance running. To some extent these are the lucky ones who have benefited from

what we can call either 'transferable skills' or 'invisible training' and their endurance training as adults is in some ways simplified.

For others, the pathway may be less gilded as we have to play catch-up for the skills that have not been so well embedded in earlier years. The general guidelines for practising these sorts of drills include:

- Try to focus on two or three key movement points on each drill; any more than

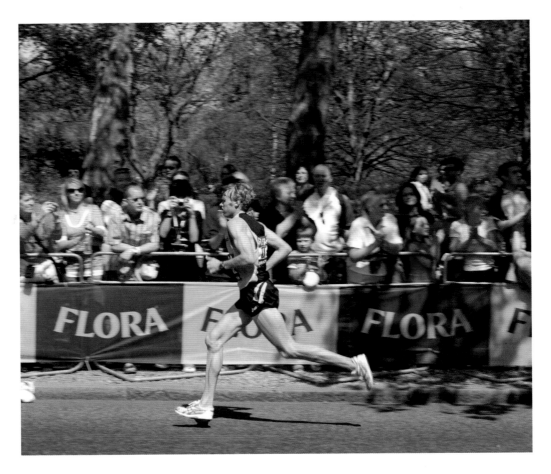

A great example of a flowing stride maintained in the marathon's final mile.

this and it is hard to give due concentration to what you are trying to achieve.

- Do each drill for about 8–10 seconds, regardless of how many reps you do in this time or what amount of ground you cover. Again, this is related to concentration levels and also to avoid any signs of fatigue creeping into the movement pattern and compromising whatever is your best attempt at it.
- Two or three reps per drill will be enough to help embed the technique; do on both left and right sides where applicable.
- Don't do the drills after a long run or hard session when you will already be fatigued, but after a comfortable-paced run of about 40–45 minutes they should be able to be carried out efficiently.
- Do a thorough warm-up before doing these drills in order to avoid doing challenging movements or positions without preparing the muscles and joints accordingly.

There is often an element of self-consciousness that many distance runners will have to overcome to do these drills, particularly if they are being performed on your own, away from a track-based group, where these drills will be seen as normal behaviour.

Whatever your actual level of movement skill, you will only be able to do the drills as well as your overall strength and conditioning allows, so there is a substantial tie-in between these elements of supplementary training. The current trend seems to be that core strength and core stability are now a part of many runners' training, particularly women runners, whereas the movement training is much more rarely integrated. It is true that you will find runners up to a fairly high level, certainly women well under 3 hours in the marathon and men sub-2.30, who don't move well and don't address this in their training.

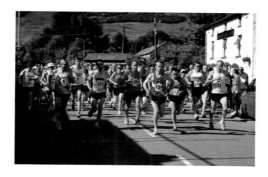

Greater movement efficiency will bring better performances in the long run.

Rather than showing that this is an optional add-on, the author suggests instead that these runners would, all things being aerobically equal, perform better if they spent some time sidelining some of the easy mileage and using the time to improve their technique.

The Running Movement Cycle

The following section is included to provide some knowledge of exactly what happens to your body when you run and therefore to provide a logical basis for the strengthening, conditioning and technical elements of training that you may carry out. The text is not a means of self-diagnosis for any injuries you may pick up. However, at some point in your running progression you are likely to suffer an injury and whoever treats the issue should apply a more detailed version of this biomechanical knowledge to address the cause of the injury. This should reduce the likelihood of its recurrence and thus link into improving your running performance.

The relationship between biomechanics and injury is specific to each body part. Overall though, poor mechanics of any body part will either increase the landing forces acting on the body, or increase the work to be done by the muscles. Both increase the stress, which – depending on the individual and the amount of running – can become excessive and cause injury. **For readers wishing to focus on the practical side without delving into the biomechanics, the relevant text is placed in bold.**

Running can be seen as a series of alternating hops from left to right leg. The ankle, knee and hip provide almost all the propulsive forces during running (apart from some upward lift from the arms). The running cycle comprises a stance phase, where one foot is in contact with the ground, while the other leg is swinging, followed by a float phase where both legs are off the ground.

The other leg then makes contact with the ground while the first leg continues to swing, followed by a second float phase. At running speeds of about 6 minutes per mile, a single running cycle will take approx 0.7 seconds, out of which each leg is only in contact with the ground for 0.22 seconds.

It is, not surprisingly, **during the stance phase that the greatest risk of injury arises**, as forces are acting on the body, muscles are active to control these forces, and joints are being loaded.

Two Sub-Phases of Stance

The first sub-phase is between 'initial contact' (IC) and 'mid-stance' (MS). IC is when the foot makes the first touch with the ground. MS is when the ankle and knee are at their maximum flexion angle. **This is the 'absorption' or the 'braking' phase. The body is going through a controlled landing; the knee and ankle flex and the foot rolls in to absorb impact forces.** At this point, the leg is storing elastic energy in the tendons and connective tissue within the muscles.

The second sub-phase is between MS and 'toe-off' (TO). **TO is the point where the foot leaves the ground. The period between MS and TO is known as the 'propulsion' phase.** The ankle, knee and hip all extend to push the body up and forwards, using the elastic energy stored during the absorption phase.

This is an efficient way for the body to work. **The more 'free' recoil energy it can draw from the bounce of the tendons, the less it has to make or to draw on from its muscle stores.** Research shows that at least half of the elastic energy comes from the Achilles and foot tendons – a reminder of how important the lower leg is to running efficiency.

Ankle, Knee and Hip Mechanics

At IC, the ankle will be slightly dorsiflexed, around 10 degrees; the knee will be flexed at 30–40 degrees and the hip flexed at about 50 degrees relative to the trunk (a fully extended hip is at 0 degrees when the midline of the thigh and the midline of the body form a straight line through the centre of the pelvis). The further forwards the trunk leans, the greater the hip flexion. Prior to IC, the hip is already extending (the leg is moving backwards) and so the foot at IC is moving back towards the hips. **If the gluteal-hamstrings are not actively pulling the foot backwards prior to IC, then the foot contact will be too far ahead of the hips** and the braking forces on the leg are increased.

During the absorption phase, the angles of flexion change. This ankle and knee flexion is coordinated to absorb the vertical landing forces on the body, which at distance running speeds are about two to three times bodyweight. This is why **eccentric strength in the calf and quadriceps muscles is required to control the knee and ankle joints, otherwise the knee and ankle would collapse or rotate inwards.** In fact, the quadriceps and calf muscles are at their most active between

IC and MS to help control the braking forces. The hip continues to extend through the absorption phase of stance.

During the propulsion phase the ankle and knee motions progress. The ankle is plantarflexed and the knee has re-extended. The hip continues to move. **Thus during the second half of the stance phase the ankle, knee and hip combine in a triple extension movement to provide propulsion upwards and forwards.** The calf, quadriceps, hamstring and gluteal activity during the propulsion phase is less than during the absorption phase, because the propulsion energy comes mainly from the recoil of elastic energy stored during the first half of stance.

The role of the muscles therefore is to control the joint positions, creating stiffness in the leg system that allows the tendons to lengthen and then recoil.

During the swing phase between TO and IC the knee and hip flex to maximum flexion and then re-extend prior to IC, with the ankle dorsiflexing.

Good runners will follow these move-ment patterns. It is essential that the ankle and knee can quickly control the braking forces and create a stable leg system to allow the tendons to maximize their recoil power. This is where good technique is vital. Too much upwards bounce will increase the land-ing forces, putting greater stress on the joints and requiring more muscle force to control. Runners need to learn to bounce along and not up, by taking quick, light steps.

It is also important to bring the foot back prior to IC using active hip extension, as this reduces braking forces and time needed for the absorption phase. Good strength in the gluteals, hamstrings, quadriceps and calf muscles will help runners to achieve this.

In summary, **excessive braking forces can contribute to injury. The correct movement patterns of the hip, knee and ankle combined** **with correct activation and strength of the major leg muscles will help control braking forces** during running and result in a more efficient action using tendon elastic energy and minimizing landing forces.

Pelvis and Trunk Mechanics

The angle of the pelvis from the side view is called the anterior–posterior tilt (A–P tilt), with a positive angle describing a tilt down towards the front.

At IC the trunk will be flexed forwards slightly and there is an A–P tilt. During the absorption phase from IC to MS, trunk flexion increases while the A–P tilt remains stable. **This slight forwards flexing of the trunk during the braking phase helps to maintain the body's forward horizontal momentum. Gluteals, hamstrings, abdominals and erec-tor spinae (stabilizing muscles in the back) are all active to control the trunk and pelvis during the absorption phase.**

During the propulsion phase the trunk re-extends to the initial position at IC. The A–P tilt will increase in line with the exten-sion. This slight shift in the anterior tilt of the pelvis helps to direct the propulsion forces of the leg horizontally. If the pelvis were in neutral, the triple extension of ankle, knee and hip would be directed more vertically.

In summary, a slight forwards lean and anterior pelvic tilt is thought efficient for running. Too much forwards lean may suggest that the posterior chain muscles (hamstrings gluteal–erector spinae) are not strong enough and this may increase the strain on the hamstrings and back during the running action. Too upright a posture may encourage vertical movement, which will increase land-ing forces.

Too much A–P tilt between IC and MS suggests that the gluteals and abdominals do not have the strength to control the pelvis adequately during landing and/or may indicate

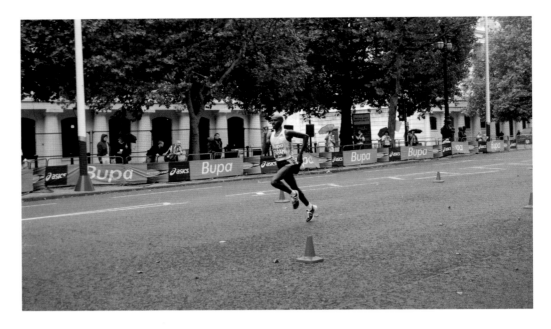

A slight forwards lean in an upright posture gains the most effective forwards velocity.

incorrect quadriceps activation and reduced hip flexibility. Excessive A–P tilt during the propulsion phases is normally associated with tight hip flexors and inadequate range of motion during hip extension. This will reduce the power of the drive from the hip and encourage a compensatory reliance on lumbar extension.

In general, a poor trunk position or lack of pelvic stability is likely to reduce the efficiency of the running action, creating extra load on the leg muscles or increasing stress through the lumbar spine and pelvis. Any of these negative factors can increase the likelihood of injury.

From the rear view the pelvic angle shows a lateral tilting, with a negative angle meaning the pelvis is tilted down towards the swing leg side. The trunk undergoes a lateral flexion with a positive angle meaning the trunk is leaning down towards the stance leg side. At faster running speeds, the lateral tilt will be bigger. There is a slight trunk lateral movement to counterbalance the pelvic tilting.

The pelvis and trunk during stance phase should be stable and provide balance. The gluteus medius muscles (abductors) are important in providing lateral stability – their contraction before and during the absorption phase prevents the hip from dropping down too far to the swing leg side. The muscles will be acting eccentrically to prevent this.

An excessive or uncontrolled pelvic tilt increases the forces through the lumbar and sacroiliac joints and forces the knee of the stance leg to rotate internally, which in turn may increase the pronation forces on the ankle. **It is possible to see a correlation between excessive pronation and excessive pelvic tilting in runners and it is a good illustration of** how one unstable link in the biomechanical chain can have an adverse knock-on effect and increase the risk of injury.

Foot Mechanics

The outwards and inwards roll of the foot during running are called supination and pronation. This rolling action is normal and healthy. It is only excessive pronation or supination that leads to injury.

At IC the foot is in a supinated position, with the rear foot inverted. During the absorption phase, the ankle is dorsiflexing, which naturally also causes the foot to pronate. **Pronation actually allows the foot to be flexible and to absorb the impact forces of landing.**

At around mid-stance the foot begins to supinate. **This moving of the foot into a more rigid position allows for a stronger push-off and more efficient recoil through the foot and Achilles tendon.** You can feel the difference for yourself – roll your heel and ankle inwards and your foot will feel soft and flat. Then roll your heel and ankle out; your foot should feel strong with an arch.

Pronation and supination both involve three-dimensional movements of the heel, ankle and tibia, which makes them very difficult to measure. The most commonly used approach is to measure the range of motion of the rear foot during the stance phase, representing the pronation and supination movement patterns. The normal trend is for the inversion (inwards-facing) angle and the eversion (outwards-facing) angles to be around 5–10 degrees.

However, foot mechanics are highly complex and are just one part of the overall picture, intertwined with what the rest of the body is doing. **Do not be rushed into deciding about the need for orthotics based solely on a visual reading of rear foot movement.**

An excessive supinator will typically land in the inverted position and then remain inverted during the stance phase. This means that they will lose out on the shock-absorbing benefits of the normal pronation movements. **Excessive supinators tend to suffer from injuries to the lateral knee and hip, and can also be prone to stress fractures**, because of the higher repetitive impact forces they incur.

If a runner spends too long in pronation, the foot will not be in a strong position to assist push-off during the propulsion phase, so the lower leg muscles will have to work harder. If the runner pronates too far or too quickly, the rotation forces acting on the tibia and knee joints may lead to problems. **Excessive pronators tend to suffer from anterior knee pain, medial tibial stress syndrome, Achilles and foot soft-tissue injuries.**

Upper Body and Arm Mechanics

The main function of the upper body and arm action is to provide balance and promote efficient movement. The arms and trunk move to oppose the forwards drive of the legs. During the braking phase, the arms and trunk produce a propulsive force and during the propulsion phase the arms and trunk combine to produce a braking force. The advantage of the out-of-phase actions of the arms and trunk is that they reduce the braking effect on the body and so conserve forwards momentum.

As the right knee drives up and through in front of the body, the left arm and shoulder move forwards – counteracting the knee motion and thereby helping to reduce rotation forces through the body during the whole movement cycle. Although the legs are much heavier than the arms, the shoulders are wider than the hips, so the arms are well-positioned for their job of counterbalancing the leg rotation. This may explain why female runners use a slightly wider or rotating arm action to compensate for their narrower shoulders and lighter upper body.

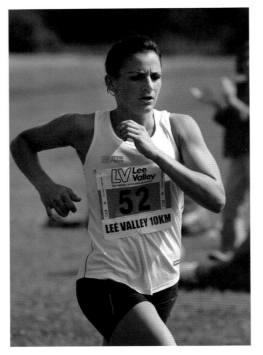

The normal arm action during distance running involves shoulder extension to pull the elbow straight back; then, as the arm comes forwards, the hand will move slightly across the body.

The arm action has more to do with running efficiency than with injury prevention directly. A good arm action needs to be encouraged to counterbalance lower-limb forces, which may in turn help to reduce injury. **The arm action also contributes a little to the vertical lift during the propulsion phase, which may help the runner to be more efficient, thus reducing the work done by the legs.**

LEFT: Focus on keeping the upper body relaxed in a race's later, fatiguing stages.

BELOW: Concentrate on relaxing tight muscle groups to maintain good form as the fatigue builds up.

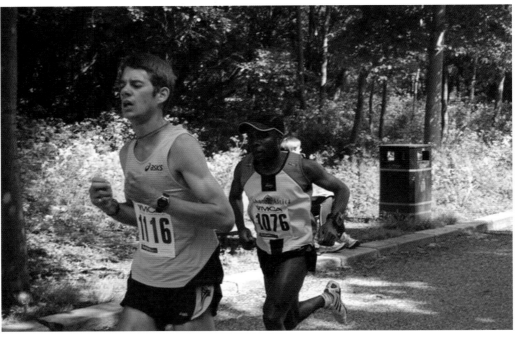

Barefoot Running

One of the recent hot topics is the supposed merits of barefoot running. The argument, simplified, is along the lines of:

- Many runners' feet are poorly conditioned for endurance training, a combination of the sedentary lifestyle most people now lead, combined with the highly overprotective cushioned heavy training shoes now produced. Using our weakened feet to do extensive road running (or, in most cases, an even more unforgiving surface, pavement running), we just compound our weaknesses, running inefficiently and becoming injured.
- Our ancient ancestors were hunter-gatherers, apparently living a quasi-endurance lifestyle by chasing animals just to keep themselves alive. They did this barefoot.
- Certain types of shoes are now available to educate our feet muscles and tendons to replicate more closely this natural movement and by doing selected bouts of barefoot running on suitable surfaces we can assist this process.

Supporters of this argument often quote the legendary Ethiopian, Abebe Bikila, who won the Olympic marathons in 1960 and 1964 without shoes, and the nationalized British runner of the 1980s, Zola Budd, who also ran barefoot in her heyday, having toughened her feet from infancy in rural South Africa. However, the overwhelming majority of elite long-distance runners, close to 100 per cent, do use training shoes even on soft surfaces and when poor young East African runners are trying to make a breakthrough in their training approach they will clamour for running shoes if they cannot otherwise afford them.

Whilst all the comments about our weakened feet sound sensible, the allusion to our supposed ancestral endurance lifestyle is somewhat inaccurate, in that prehistoric man hunted in short, sharp bursts, which, even if they did last many hours or even days to catch the hunted animal, were not endurance running in any sustained form, but a series of unstructured shorter bursts with long breaks. For avoidance of doubt, this hunting was done on much softer surfaces than pavements and tarmac.

One of the most authoritative voices on this subject is leading British podiatrist Clifton Bradeley, formerly a sub-4-minute miler who has spent the last twenty-five years professionally working with sports people's feet and movement patterns. His view is, quite simply, if we were meant to run barefoot we would have been doing it a long time ago: 'The notion that the caveman would run a barefoot marathon every day to gather food is not correct, we evolved to hunt as a group at speed over short distances.'

As for forefoot running, and similar 'schools' of supposedly optimum running movement such as Chi and POSE running, again Bradeley is very cautious. Eighty per cent of runners run heel to toe. The view is that by trying to alter this gait through specific drills or by purchasing special equipment, Newton shoes for example, we massively increase our risk of injury. This is because of a concept called asymmetry.

Years of research and practice has convinced Bradeley that the key to efficient and successful running performance comes from the pelvic position and its relation to the upper and lower body. Hip height and leg length discrepancies can play havoc over long periods of sustained running on flat, hard surfaces as the body tries to compensate, causing excess pronation and postural changes; '95 per cent of non-traumatic sports injuries can be put down to body asymmetry,' says Bradeley, who believes that effective shoe design and the use of orthotics are the only way to control this effectively over the long term. For example, in Japan, 283 elite athletes had their foot strike recorded by high-speed video at the 15km mark of a half-marathon. A large majority, 75 per cent, were heel strikers. Less than 2 per cent (just four out of the 283) were forefoot strikers. Some further points to consider about barefoot running:

- Every person is individual and what works for one does not work for all. Not all runners need to strike on their forefoot to be the most efficient runners. For many runners at their normal training speeds, rearfoot striking is actually the preferred manner of running.
- Trying to make someone who is naturally a rearfoot striker into a forefoot striker may injure them.
- A runner who is a rearfoot striker at 10:00 minutes per mile pace may be a forefoot striker at 5:00 minutes per mile pace. Remember: running speed changes the foot-strike pattern. For endurance runners this may prompt a revisiting of the notion of a universal 'best practice' model. A top-level 1,500m runner will race at a speed not that far removed from their full speed – perhaps 14 seconds per 100m with their maximum sprint speed typically just under 12 seconds per 100m. The comparable level at a marathon would be about 18 or 19 seconds per 100m, so the biomechanics and need for power versus economy of stride are different. The same principles will apply to runners of less exalted standard, maybe even more so because they are likely to have a greater differential between their maximum speed and their long-distance race pace.

- Running barefoot strengthens the postural muscles in the feet and lower leg, if these have previously been neglected by under-use and/or heavily cushioned shoes.
- Running barefoot/minimalist increases proprioceptive (spatial) awareness and balance. This should result in a slight improvement of running efficiency.
- Running barefoot/minimalist forces a change in mechanics to adapt to the forces on the feet.
- There are as yet no clinical trials that show an effect of barefoot running for a prolonged period of time.
- There are currently no research studies that prove that wearing traditional running shoes increases injuries or that barefoot/minimalist running reduces injuries (and vice versa).

In summary, if you are considering switching to a more 'minimal' running shoe, do some further reading around the subject and ensure you follow a gradual transition programme.

KEY POINTS

- A technically efficient runner will on average be less likely to pick up injuries than an inefficient runner.
- Consider the link between your strength and conditioning and your capacity to maintain your optimum running movement.
- Heel strikers do not need to force themselves to become forefoot strikers to become decent long-distance runners.
- The barefoot running debate is not clear cut and leading podiatrists are cautious on fully embracing it.

CHAPTER 8

FLEXIBILITY, STRENGTH AND PHYSICAL CONDITIONING

The contents of this chapter are linked to the detail of Chapter 7, relating to the biomechanics of running movement. To move optimally at your target running speeds, you need to be flexible enough, strong enough and powerful enough to do so without becoming injured, while using as little energy as possible.

Flexibility

This is invariably one of the hot topics in any discussion on injury prevention and running technique. Despite various pieces of research in recent decades there is not yet any totally consistent approach within the sport on the merits of static stretching for endurance running.

If we look at the range of flexibility needed for long-distance running it is clearly a smaller range of movement than is needed for 400m running, which is itself a narrower range of movement than is required for 110m hurdles. Of course, if we watch a mid-pack distance runner, particularly in the later stages of a race, we may see a cramped, shuffling style showing limited range of movement, particularly from the waist down. This will be visibly a very different movement from how Mo Farah will blast round the final lap of a 10,000m race in 53 seconds. So we would make the easy, and at least partly correct, judgement that the slower runner lacked flexibility and the

simple recommendation would be 'do more stretching', or, in some cases, 'start doing some stretching'.

In this context of relevant flexibility, each muscle has an optimal length whereby on contraction it can produce its maximum power – this is its 'torque'. Beyond this point, increased flexibility – manifested in greater muscle length – reduces power and thus negates performance. In terms of injury prevention, it is strength more than flexibility in a muscle that is more relevant. The muscle's eccentric strength is its capacity to resist lengthening and the length/power balance is what is important in the muscles used in running.

That said, many runners may indeed have limited flexibility for what is needed for their events at their target pace, and particularly veteran runners where the natural default is to experience a reducing range of movement with increased age (see Chapter 6).

When warming up before a race, bear in mind that there is no valid evidence that static stretching in the warm-up phase either assists better performance or prevents injury. Indeed, if you do a significantly different routine from your training session warm-up, you may actually worsen your performance by putting your muscles through unaccustomed movements and with body temperature going down rather than up. This race-specific scenario is mentioned because training sessions may, in reality, be slightly rushed, whereas the extra

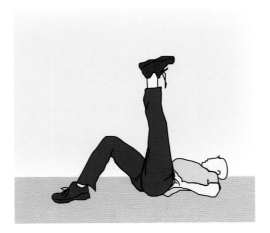

This leg extension drill works the hamstrings, hip flexors, gluteals and abdominals.

tion. There is at least medical support to actively avoid restricting one's flexibility. In *The Complete Guide to Stretching*, physiotherapist Chris Norris states 'When the full range [of extensibility and elasticity] does not occur, the muscle can shorten permanently and alter the function of a joint.'

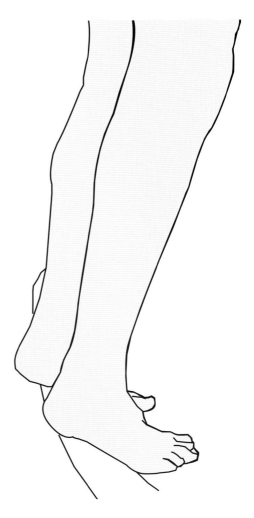

time that a runner may have allowed to arrive at a race venue may lead into the thinking that 'more is better'. For the range of movement deployed in a race of 10km or further, it is unlikely that any additional static stretching will be needed. Your 'fit for purpose' state can be achieved by a build-up of easy and steady running, some skipping for both height and length, and some faster strides at about your target race pace or slightly faster.

The above notes of caution should not be confused with a stretching programme that has been advised by a medical practitioner, where specific areas are shown to lack the required range of movement for the runner's purpose, resulting in an injury.

In researching this book, the author checked the advice on stretching in other running publications and there is no particular regime that is consistently backed up by research. Some writers suggest, simplistically, that it is unlikely to do any harm to at least maintain your range of movement, and combine this with what seems logical based on observa-

Calf raises, using a suitable level of resistance for each runner, are a key element in injury prevention to the calf, Achilles and even the knee.

Strength/Strength-Endurance and Power

The English Institute of Sport, the pan-sports agency that helps to prepare elite athletes in more than thirty sports, describes its approach to strength and conditioning as based on 'optimizing the body's force, power and velocity capabilities specific for the athlete and the event'.

In applying this to endurance runners, there are some proven research findings:

- In 1999 controlled tests showed that 5km/10km runners who completed a nine-week programme of explosive strength drills improved performance more than those that did no such resistance training. The improvements were shown not to have been derived from additional advances in either VO_2 max or lactate threshold compared to the control group, but from progress in running economy and neuromuscular adaptations.
- In 2000, further research showed that improved running speeds were based on achieving greater ground forces, and that the limiting factor in this is the time available to exert one's force, rather than the maximum force itself. Simplifying, it is more about power (the speed at which strength is utilized), than maximum strength itself.

The key to developing power for running is one's elasticity. Only about 50 per cent of the energy produced by oxygen during running aerobically is actually used in fuelling the muscles' movement forwards. About 5–10 per cent is used in shock absorption and about 10–15 per cent is needed to overcome air resistance. About 40 per cent is stored within the muscles and is available for their elastic capability. Of this 40 per cent, half is channelled below the knee to the Achilles tendon and the arches of the feet.

Moving from the scientist's outlook to that of the endurance coach, George Gandy, current UK Athletics Endurance Head Coach, describes the need 'to develop strength for force in the propulsive muscles and for tolerance of stresses by equally attuned non-propulsive elements. Sufficient freedom of joint movements must also be ensured so as best to apply these forces, and enough specific endurance to allow the process to be repeated as often and as quickly as required.'

So, in practice, and without the benefit of an expert strength and conditioning coach to give you an individualized programme, do try to focus on development of power rather than strength itself so that the challenge is specific to what your running progress requires.

Bear in mind that this is very much a means to an end and you are just trying to make yourself 'fit for purpose'. A shot putter or sprint hurdler might expect to see some direct links between what they can achieve in weight training and how this translates to their target event, whereas a long-distance runner would be less likely to see such a clear link.

However, every runner is only as strong as their weakest link. We can illustrate this by two examples, both fairly typical in the current running environment. First, a male, mid-thirties, who has played rugby and cricket through school, university and at club level, with regular coached training sessions in both sports. Fairly new to any endurance sport, although he also keeps up a simple weekly gym session from what he recalls of his rugby conditioning, he is a 45-minute 10km runner and wishes to break 3.45 for a marathon. So he is not yet looking to run especially quickly, and he brings a historically well-conditioned frame to his current running level.

Contrast this with a female of similar age, who was never involved with sport at school but who has belatedly found her niche in distance running, now covering 60 miles weekly and looking to break 37 minutes for 10km. To do this, she will need to be doing some training and racing at significantly faster than her target 10km time, at maybe 5 minutes 30 seconds per mile, or just over 80 seconds per lap of a 400m track. If she has no conditioning background, either for running or another sport, then her aerobic and cardiovascular level may be well in advance of the underlying strength and she carries a high injury risk. The classic analogy is that of a motor car's chassis and engine. Our hypothetical ex-rugby player needs to build up his engine within a strong chassis, whereas the speedy woman needs to ensure her chassis is strong enough to withstand the velocity that her engine makes her capable of generating and sustaining.

As guidelines on how to fit strength and conditioning (S+C) sessions into your running programme, consider the following:

- Even at very high level there is not universal agreement amongst coaches and athletes on how close to the competition phase one should maintain an S+C routine. But bear in mind the overarching principle of specificity – and doing a set of lunges, step-ups and dead lifts on a Tuesday before a half-marathon on the Sunday certainly won't contribute to a new PB on the day (though it might make a contribution towards making you more robust to tackle further training once you have recovered from the half-marathon). The typical trend would – as logic suggests – involve more frequent S+C in the general training phase and less in the specific event preparation. This would be broadly the opposite to how the running load changes.
- Try to avoid doing an S+C session within about 4 hours either before or after a running session if at all possible. There is a theory that this causes an 'interference effect', which results in both the aerobic and the strength session being somewhat reduced in their effect. There have been numerous research projects to try to establish a clear rationale on how to manage this, but the results are not conclusive. It is acknowledged that in reality when people sometimes have just one training window in a day, the sessions may have to follow one another. And indeed many very good club groups have a regular structure of doing an easy or steady run and then proceeding directly to some sort of strength/strength-endurance session. There is a logic that if a strength session is to be done at a challenging level of resistance, being fatigued at the start from a tough aerobic session will not enable you to perform as you would wish in the strength session, and one would not find good athletes going from a tough interval or threshold session to a meaningful resistance session – though they may do so later in the same day.
- Do allow at least 48 hours between conditioning sessions. If they are challenging enough to be of benefit, then they will be enough that you need at least a day of recovery and absorption before taking up the challenge again.

Pilates

In recent years the growth in popularity of Pilates, and its application for distance running, has brought it into consideration as part of many runners' conditioning programmes. In the UK one of its leading proponents in athletics has been Joe Mills, a former national 1,500m champion and sub-4-minute miler who now practises in the Canadian high-performance

This focuses on lower back, hamstrings and gluteals.

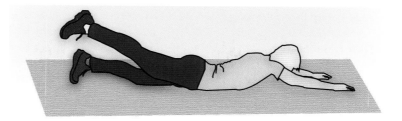

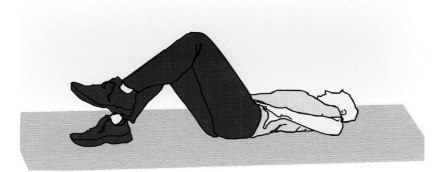

For strength and stability in the abdominals, gluteals and quadriceps.

Strength and balancing exercise for lower back and abdominals.

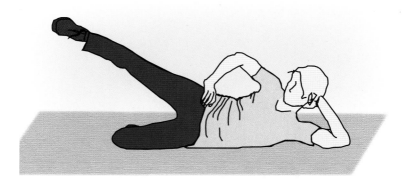

system. He summarizes the aspects where Pilates can bring benefit as follows:

- **Ineffective muscle use** Specifically, losing the correct and optimum balance between the mobilizing muscles and the stabilizing muscles.
- **Faulty recruitment patterns** Muscles

work in groups to achieve the optimal and most economical movement patterns and typical sedentary lifestyles tend to result in deviating from the optimum. So runners will adopt inefficient recruitment patterns in their running and these become embedded as the norm unless something is done to remedy them.

- **Neutral pelvis and spine** These form the body's axis from which all movement stems, so the two aspects above need to be rooted in a strong, well-aligned spine and pelvis. This is why all Pilates sessions start with the requirement to establish, and be able to feel, what comprises neutral.

- **Joints** Once one has lost ideal posture and muscle balance, the impact forces through activities such as running will not be so fully absorbed through the central – and strongest – section of the affected joints. Over time, this is likely to lead to excessive wear and tear around the joint, with ensuing higher risk of injury. For the

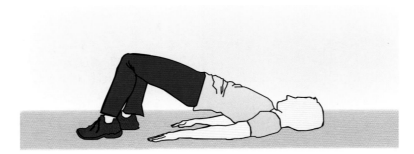

The much-used Bridge works the back, abdominals and gluteals.

Abdominals, gluteals and lower back are worked in single leg extensions.

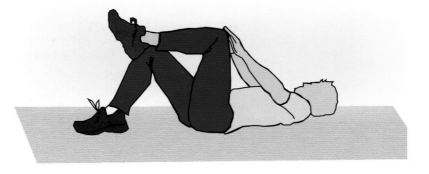

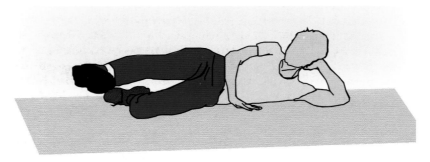

Hip-flexor muscles are tested in this side stretch, as are abdominals.

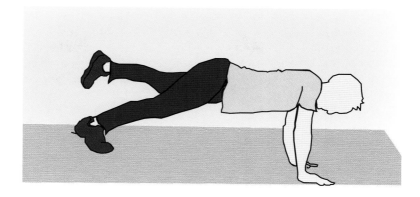

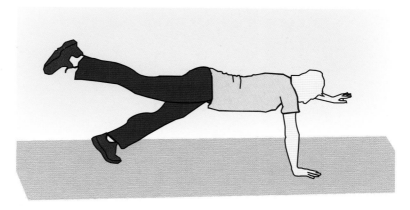

The famous Plank and its variations engage the back, gluteals and abdominals.

runner, this will typically relate to knees, hips and ankles.

- **Breathing** There is an intrinsic link between the muscular efficiency around the core, which is of course where all the respiratory organs are located, and the 'quality' of the breathing itself. As endurance-running performance is related to the amount of oxygen taken in and used around the body, breathing inefficiencies will impact adversely on performance.

Do be aware that Pilates may not meet all of a runner's strength and conditioning needs, depending on where each runner sits on the balance between strength and endur-

ance. Also, many drills that one encounters in a Pilates session have been absorbed or transferred across to other regimes that may be called 'core strength', 'core stability' or body conditioning'. So, for example, many runners will do exercises commonly called 'Crab', 'Plank' or 'Bridge' without ever having attended a Pilates session. But if your core is fit for purpose you probably are not too concerned about who 'invented' the system into which you are tapping.

Pilates can therefore benefit the runner through low threshold recruitment of the deep abdominal muscles, improved posture, efficient breathing and the importance of correct neutral alignment during functional movement. It is possible that a regular set of drills rooted in Pilates principles, combined with structured hill-running sessions, may meet most, or indeed all, of your conditioning to make you fit for purpose for your running goals.

Theory Into Practice

All of this material about torque, energy return, mobilizers and stabilizers might leave you wondering what level of sophistication needs to go into your own sessions. Be assured that there is a large amount you can do that may well be familiar from general circuit training.

As an example, the large and successful Birmingham University endurance squad, whose recent athletic alumni include World and Olympic marathon runner Dave Webb and World 1,500m silver medallist Hannah England, has a regular weekly circuits session based around the following. The structure is that three sets of all drills are done, with the effort versus recovery split being about 25 seconds of work with 10 seconds of recovery and transition. It is worth noting that the abdominals have a variety of drills so that there is a more widespread development of muscles

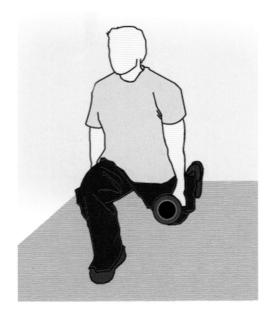

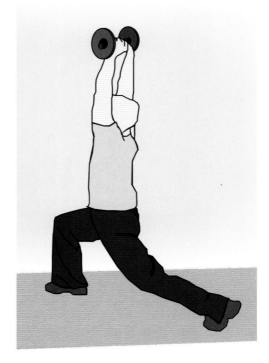

Lunges, with slightly varying positions and grades of resistance, condition the gluteals, quadriceps and hip flexors.

around the core area, and not just an unhelpful isolated focus on a six-pack surrounded by relatively weaker muscles. The duration of the session is designed to give a suitable balance of strength endurance for endurance runners, so is not an aerobic training stimulus.

Hip-flexor circuits:

- high knees;
- split jumps;
- single leg squats, left and right;
- lying down on side, side leg raises, left and right;
- lunges front;
- lunges backwards.

Abdominals circuits:

- sit-ups over knees;
- feet together, side touches;
- high reaches;
- sit-ups hands to opposite knee;
- double feet up and out;
- buttock to ankle touches;
- leg shoot.

Some similar benefits are achieved by what the aforementioned Gandy developed over many years at Loughborough University, which has been a hub of British elite endurance running for nearly forty years. The conditioning programme is perhaps simpler than might be expected, given the scientific talk that underpins it. It includes:

- bounding;
- press-ups;
- squat thrusts;
- chinnies (or chin-ups);
- hip thrusts;
- skipping;
- rope climb;
- bent leg sit-ups;
- step-ups onto a 30cm step/box.

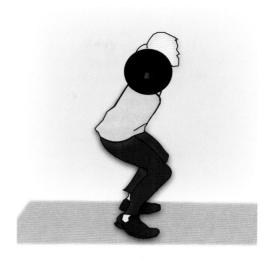

The squat is the classic resistance exercise for all-over conditioning. It engages the gluteals, quadriceps and hamstrings. It is fine for beginners to use bodyweight or very low extra weight. A straight back, correct positioning and movement are essential to reduce injury risk.

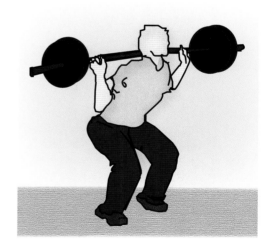

This advanced drill progresses the basic squat into an explosive power-based movement.

In addition, for a more advanced challenge, box jumping and rebounds can be added for a greater plyometric challenge, although this should be done only by athletes robust enough to do so, as the injury risk is higher.

The structure of the session would be along the lines of thirty circuits of 30 seconds (maximum), with a maximum of 30 seconds recovery/transition, so a broadly similar strength-endurance focus as the Birmingham option. Nearly all of these can be readily carried out in one's own home if a gym is not always accessible, although rope climbs will only be found in the more idiosyncratically furnished living rooms.

Hills for All-Round Training Conditioning

The following paragraphs show how hill training can be used to cover these training bases without necessarily being rooted in the finer points of exercise science.

Two examples of high achievers using short hills as their means of developing running power are Eamonn Martin, former UK Record holder at 10,000m (still third on our all-time lists) and the last British male winner of the London Marathon, with his trademark sprint finish in 1993 (on his debut too), and Rob Denmark, Commonwealth 5,000m champion and the last British-born man to make the Top Eight in Olympic and World Championships finals at 5,000m. Both of these runners had big sprint finishes to back up their huge aerobic capacity, yet both did fairly simple regimes of general conditioning exercises that most school PE teachers or a basic-level personal trainer could advise on. Martin has described how he did some press-ups and sit-ups first thing in the morning while he waited for the kettle to boil, and indeed when in his later years the commercial returns on his running

freed up a little extra time to start on a more robust weightlifting programme, there was not a discernible improvement in running performance.

However, the major conditioning element that these athletes managed to gain from their running programme was the strength and strength-endurance derived from short and quite steep hill repetitions. Both Martin and Denmark – and indeed other high achievers from the area around Basildon, Essex, that has been a stronghold of endurance running down the years – used a particular hill that took about 25 seconds to run up at high intensity, with a turnaround and jog back recovery of about 45 seconds. If you analyse the movement patterns involved in short hill bursts, you will see that they challenge and develop the key muscle groups used in some of the classic conditioning drills such as lunges, step-ups and half squats.

KEY POINTS

- Dynamic flexibility drills can have a big role in making your range of movement fit for purpose.
- Focus on power (speed applied to strength) as an essential tool to improve performance.
- Pilates has considerable benefits and is worth including as part of a conditioning plan.
- Simple but diverse and progressive circuit sessions offer a practical and enjoyable way to make gains in power and strength endurance.
- Use hills as a multi-purpose training option. Short hills will keep a focus on the strength/speed endurance/strength-endurance factors.

CHAPTER 9

NUTRITION AND HYDRATION

Overview

'There should be no conflict between eating for health and eating for performance. The sound basis for a successful sporting diet is one based on healthy eating principles and a balanced approach.' That is the official UK Athletics introduction to its nutrition module for coaches. It provides a further eighteen pages that should cover nearly all that a coach or athlete really needs to know for their events. At first glance it seems strange that such a bland overview can be consistent with the ever-increasing volume of books about sports nutrition.

But before we look any further at what foods (or 'nutritional strategies', as we now seem obliged to describe them) may help your running, let's use some elite coaches' and athletes' wisdom for context. England Athletics' National Coach Mentor for Endurance, himself an Olympic athlete with a Masters in Sports Science, advised coaches 'a good square meal backed up with quality snacking, breakfast and lunch usually provide 99 per cent of what you need', whilst also seeking to see how the other 1 per cent might be acquired.

'I eat the same as my wife, only more of it,' said Olympic 10,000m medallist Brendan Foster in his autobiography, written at his peak in the late 1970s. The book does not enlighten us on Mrs Foster's meal plans. Fellow Geordie Olympic medallist Charlie Spedding writes in his book of how 'I think a lot of newcomers

were hoping they could be able to eat themselves into peak physical condition ... there were various fad foods and supplements and I was often asked if this or that food would improve performance.' He does observe, tongue in cheek, that cottage cheese must be a particularly unhelpful choice as he only ever sees obese people eating it. As a pharmacist and a meticulous planner, there is no suspicion that Spedding had an unduly casual approach – he simply evaluated its relative importance. His track record – he is still the English record holder at marathon with 2.08.33 – suggests his judgement was spot on.

The author has spent hundreds of hours in coaching seminars and conferences with some of the best in the endurance business and, almost without exception, the coaches' presentations and ideas will not have nutrition at their heart and yet, invariably, questions from the floor will focus on nutrition far more than the presenting coach would have planned. Also, the more experienced the coaches and athletes in attendance, the more they will keep nutrition where it belongs – it underpins running improvement, but it certainly does not deliver it. For that, we have to leave the kitchen table and head out for some running.

Or, put another way, if you train very sensibly but eat a far from optimum diet, you should still run close to your full potential. But if you train very haphazardly whilst following a nutritionally perfect plan for a healthy sporting life, you will not perform well as a distance runner. Indeed, research for this book came up with the information contained in the table presented here, and bear in mind that in each case the book is written by a proven high-level coach or sports scientist.

So, an interesting scenario in which out of some 2,200 pages of the most influential guidance on long-distance running, about 4 per cent is allocated to nutrition and hydration other than the specific carbohydrate needs of a marathon. The rationale here is not that the writers don't care about nutrition. Far from it, but rather their expertise is based on a holistic approach to training people they coach and the most significant part of this whole is the running itself. Similarly, these coaches and

Pages Allocated to Nutrition and Hydration in Influential Books on Long-Distance Running

Title	Total Page Number	Total Pages on Diet inc Hydration and Electrolytes	Pages on Carbo-Loading Diet	Pages Describing Overemphasis on Diet	Net Pages on Diet
Tim Noakes, *Lore of Running*	750 (sic)	47	7	3	37
Pfitzinger and Douglas, *Advanced Marathoning*	210	16	4	1	11
AAA, *Runners' Guide*	190	10	2	1	7
Bruce Tulloh, *Running at 40+*	190	10	1	1	8
Jack Daniels, *Running Formula*	270	0	0	0	0
Cliff Temple, *Marathon, Cross-Country and Road*	190	12	6	1	5
Dionisio Alonso, *Spanish Marathon Techniques*	280	18	5	2	11
David Costill, *Scientific Approach to Distance Running*	130	9	4	0	5

authors will be aware of the importance of the mental aspect of running and of course the intricate world of injury treatment, but the publications on these areas, just as with nutrition, are written by those who have made these aspects, rather than coaching, their focus.

Scouring some other volumes aimed at more beginner runners, the typical proportion on nutrition and hydration is between 10 and 15 per cent. That said, it is obviously sensible to ensure as far as possible that you are covering the bases for your training and racing.

The Basic Food Groups and Requirements

Carbohydrates, proteins and fats are the three macronutrients that provide energy in a form that is necessary for survival. Alcohol is the only other source of energy, but that is not essential for survival – although you will more often hear runners saying 'I really need a pint' than they will mention a craving for some whey protein. If you are aware of the key elements of the food groups and maintain a good balance in line with your own training habits, you should be taking on board adequate fuelling for your running.

Carbohydrates are the macronutrient that we need in the largest amounts. Depending on your level of physical activity, about 50–65 per cent of your energy should come from carbohydrate. Carbohydrates are the body's main source of fuel. They:

- are easily used by the body for energy;
- are needed for the central nervous system, the kidneys, the brain and the muscles (including the heart) to function properly;

- can be stored in the muscles and liver and later used for energy;
- are important in intestinal health and waste elimination;
- are mainly found in starchy foods (like grain, rice and potatoes), fruits, milk and yoghurt. Other foods such as vegetables, beans, nuts and seeds contain carbohydrates, but in lesser amounts.

In addition, all of the tissues and cells in our body can use glucose (which is the usable form of carbohydrate after digestion) for energy.

Fibre refers to certain types of carbohydrates that our body cannot digest. These carbohydrates pass through the intestinal tract intact and help to move waste out of the body. Diets that are low in fibre have been shown to cause problems such as constipation and haemorrhoids and to increase the risk of certain types of cancers. Diets high in fibre have been shown to reduce the risk of heart disease and obesity, as well as helping to lower cholesterol. Foods high in fibre include fruits, vegetables and whole-grain products.

Depending on individual activity levels, between 10 and 30 per cent of calories should come from protein. Most British people get plenty of protein and easily meet this need by consuming a balanced diet. We need protein for:

- growth (especially important for children, teenagers and pregnant women);
- tissue repair;
- immune function;
- making essential hormones and enzymes ;
- energy when carbohydrate is not available;
- preserving lean muscle mass.

Protein is found in meats, poultry, fish, meat substitutes, cheese, milk, nuts, legumes and in smaller quantities in starchy foods and vegetables.

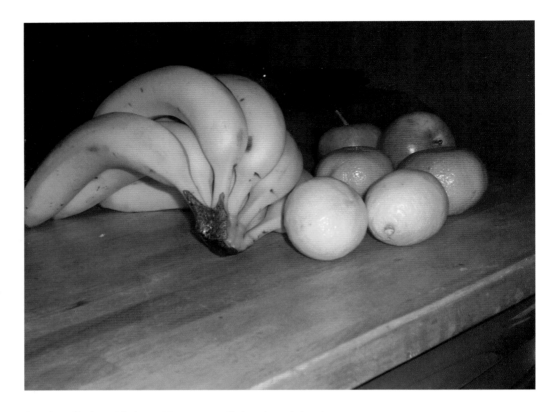

A variety of coloured fruit provides a range of minerals and vitamins.

When we eat these types of foods, our body breaks down the protein they contain into amino-acids (the building blocks of proteins). Some amino-acids are essential, which means that we need to get them from our diet, while others are non-essential because our body can make them. Protein that comes from animal sources contains all of the essential amino-acids that we need; plant sources of protein, on the other hand, do not.

Although fats have received a bad reputation for causing weight gain, some fat is essential for survival. Between about 10 and 20 per cent of calories should come from fat. We need this amount of fat for:

- normal growth and development;
- energy (fat is the most concentrated source of energy);
- absorbing certain vitamins (such as vitamins A, D, E and K);
- providing cushioning for the organs;
- maintaining cell membranes;
- providing taste, consistency and stability to foods.

Fat is found in meat, poultry, nuts, milk products, butters and margarines, oils, lard, fish, grain products and salad dressings. There are three main types of fat – saturated fat, unsaturated fat and trans-fat. Saturated fat (found in foods such as meat, butter, lard and cream) and trans-fat (found in baked goods, snack foods, fried foods and margarines) have been shown to increase the risk of heart disease. Replacing saturated and trans-fat in your diet with unsaturated fat (found in foods such as olive oil, avocados and nuts) has been shown to decrease the risk of developing heart disease.

Some Specifics for Long-Distance Runners

Post-Training Refuelling Window

When you exercise aerobically, you are running down your glycogen (carbohydrate) supplies and breaking down muscle tissues (protein, simplistically). Therefore to restore your body to its pre-training state you need to ingest a suitable quantity of carbohydrate and protein. An enzyme that is released during exercise enables your body to have a heightened capacity to absorb carbs and protein in a 30-minute window after training. A ratio of about 1g of carbohydrate and 0.25g of protein

per kg of bodyweight is shown to be the optimum to kick-start this recovery process. For most people this equates to a snack of about 300 to (for heavier runners) 400 calories of carb and protein, taken either as a solid, or as a specific sports-recovery drink.

There is evidence that a balance of whey and casein protein is the particular structure of amino-acid that helps the recovery process. Whey is the 'fast' protein that quickly enters the system to enable further protein synthesis to rebuild the muscles, whilst casein is the 'slow' protein that raises the amino-acid levels in the bloodstream to ensure this rebuilding is sustained. So – in addition to the ever-increasing range of bespoke supplements provided by the sports nutrition sector – look for foods such as bread, yoghurt, soft low-fat cheese, tea cakes or scones with a low-fat filling to fuel this snack.

Iron

It is worth giving particular focus to this mineral because it is so essential to your running performance and because it is very easy to have a low level. This will affect your

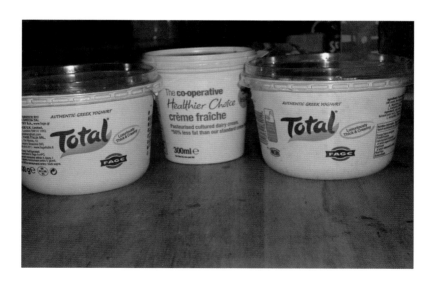

Yoghurt – an ideal mix of carbohydrate and protein for post-run refuelling.

running quite noticeably but will not necessarily be picked up in a standard GP's blood test, as this looks at what is needed for general health, which for the vast majority is a fairly sedentary lifestyle.

One needs to distinguish between iron-deficiency anaemia, which is fairly rare in endurance runners (less than 2 per cent of women and even rarer in males), and the much more prevalent earlier symptoms of non-anaemic iron deficiency that occurs in about 25–45 per cent of female runners and about 5 per cent of males. Whilst anaemia most definitely has a major adverse effect on endurance performance, the more prevalent deficiency is not conclusively shown to affect your running adversely, although most tests suggest that this is the case.

The 2011 European Athletics Federation's Endurance Conference included a keynote presentation on the subject, as an indicator of its importance. Iron is essential for red blood cell formation and thus the transportation and utilization of oxygen so is at the heart of endurance capacity for any sport. Women need almost twice as high a daily intake as men – around 15–18 milograms for women and about 8 milograms for men. The best options for iron in a normal diet include red meat, leafy green vegetables, breakfast cereals, dried fruits, pulses, nuts and seeds. What needs to be considered are habits that can restrict iron absorption, including tea and coffee drunk within 1 hour either side of eating iron, high fibre intakes and zinc or calcium supplements.

The indicator of your iron level is your ferretin count. Ferritin is a measure of the body's iron stores. Normal reference ferritin levels are 12–200ng (nanograns)/ml for women and 13–300ng/ml for men. Ferritin is not directly related to performance, but if your ferritin level falls eventually your haemoglobin and performances will decline too. Low ferritin, therefore, can be viewed as an early warning sign.

Ball-park figures suggest that training and racing performances are usually affected when ferritin levels drop below 20ng/ml, and that when those athletes increase their ferritin levels above 25ng/ml they experience a rapid turnaround in performance. Bear in mind that counts in the twenties and low thirties are very common in distance runners and this is often just the level at which your GP will not be concerned about any impact on general health, but where as a runner you may be convinced that something is not firing on all cylinders.

Low iron intake can be a problem for vegetarians and for those runners who eat red meat less than once per week. The typical high-carbohydrate, low-fat, low-cholesterol runner's diet often includes little or no red meat. Red meat contains haem iron, which is more easily absorbed than plant sources of iron.

Another factor that may tilt the balance for some runners is foot-strike haemolysis. This is the breakdown of red blood cells when the foot hits the ground. While foot-strike haemolysis is not a big problem for most runners, if you are larger than average or run high mileage on asphalt, it could be a factor.

A relatively small amount of iron is lost through sweat and urine, but if you are doing heavy training in hot, humid conditions, this iron loss may add up. More research is needed to determine the magnitude of this problem.

You can only confirm your suspicions, however, with a blood test. You should find out both your haemoglobin and serum ferritin levels. Normal haemoglobin concentration ranges from 14–18g per 100ml of blood for men, and 12–16g per 100ml of blood for women, but for an endurance athlete, the lower end of normal should be extended by about 1g per 100ml, due to our larger blood volume.

The following actions should in most cases prevent iron deficiency:

- eating 3oz (90g) of lean red meat or dark poultry a couple of times per week;
- no coffee or tea with meals (that is, within an hour before or after), because they reduce iron absorption;
- eating or drinking vitamin C-rich foods with meals to increase iron absorption.

Although these recommendations may seem like subtle changes in diet, they can have a powerful effect on your iron levels. For example, you will absorb three times as much iron from your cereal and toast if you switch from coffee to orange juice with breakfast. Iron supplements, in the form of ferrous sulphate, ferrous gluconate or ferrous fumarate, should be taken only if they are still necessary after making the recommended dietary changes.

Bodyweight

A sensitive issue for some, but it's naïve to ignore the indisputable fact that quicker runners are relatively light in bodyweight. If we remember that our maximum aerobic capacity (VO_2 max) is a bodyweight-based measurement, then the basic science indicates that if all our aerobic and cardiovascular traits stay the same but we use these traits to shift a lighter body mass, then we will go faster for a given level of effort.

Anecdotally, the author has noted that many very swift endurance runners are just not foodie types. Meals are simply refuelling for them – they eat, they start to feel full, they stop eating. These are the types who often struggle to keep their weight up when they are in heavy training and when they are injured or eventually stop serious running they stay virtually the same weight, albeit their shape and muscle tone may slacken slightly over time.

To lose 1lb (0.5kg) you need to use up some 3,500 kilocalories (kcals) more than you take in. Your running training will use up, at a weight of 10 stone (63kg), about 100kcals per mile. Broadly, pro-rata this amount if you are lighter or heavier and also note that as long as you are running mainly aerobically this figure will not vary significantly with the running pace, although of course the quicker you go the more calories per minute you use. Indeed, walking a mile uses a very similar amount of energy.

The psychology around food is a highly complex issue and not for this book. Losing a small amount of weight will not revolutionize your results. A 1kg (2.2lb) weight loss will, all other things being equal, bring about a performance improvement of between 1 and 2 per cent. But it's hard to be exact, because usually all other things are not equal. Typically, an endurance athlete losing weight will also have some sort of changes in training volume and/or training intensity and/or planning structure and/or motivation and mental focus. So if a lighter athlete is making huge progress, be aware that they are probably also improving some other performance factors to achieve this.

We can all make our personal choices on how important the extra few seconds per mile are when set against a second portion of an absolutely corking Bakewell tart. The witty expert American running writer Hal Higdon describes how after weeks of hard, purposeful training and two days of carbohydrate depletion before a marathon he is let loose on a large ice-cream sundae as he starts the loading phase. He writes that if told that each spoonful adds a minute to his marathon time, he would still carry on fuelling until he hit the excess half-hour mark. As some real broad-brush guidance, if you choose to lose some weight to aid running performance, try to adhere to the following:

- Do make it gradual – 1 kg (2.2lb) per fort-night at the maximum.
- Do ensure you stay hydrated and don't 'manipulate' weight loss through dehydra-tion.
- Do not cut back on your basic complex carbohydrate or protein needs, or elimi-nate fat from your diet. You need all of these to ensure some sort of qual-ity for your training and recovery, let alone the daily business of normal life.

Instead, cut back on the empty calories of refined carbohydrates, saturated fats and alcohol. Alcohol can be doubly villainous in that it provides 'useless' calories and also tends to reduce willpower to resist other foods.

- Try to shed the excess during the general training phase rather than the specific phase if at all possible. It's a small point, but you would be better off being fully fuelled for the event-specific phase.

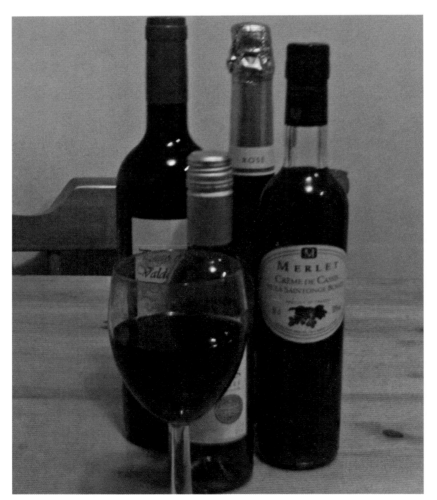

Wine is healthy in small amounts; less useful in excess.

Carbohydrate Loading
for the Marathon

As a brief summary, the traditional 'hardcore' depletion and loading diet was initially used by Scandinavian cross-country skiers in the 1960s. For the running world, it was developed by elite British marathoner and scientist Ron Hill in the late 1960s and was gradually refined and moderated in subsequent decades. The original regime comprised:

- A very long run, about 2 hours, at strong pace, seven days before a marathon.
- Three days of very minimal carbohydrate intake, with reduced running volume – this, combined with the depletion of the long run, reduced muscle and liver glycogen to very low levels, with the body crying out for carbohydrates. Weight would go down in this short phase.
- Three days of further reduced running, but fuelled with an overload of carbohydrates. The amount of calories taken in was not expressly increased, but the proportions were shifted substantially towards carbs and away from fat and protein. Weight would increase, as 4g of water are needed to be stored within the body for every 1g of glycogen. Typically, a runner would gain 2–3kg in this period, so would stand on the marathon start line maybe 1.5–2kg over normal weight. This extra baggage in the form of additional glycogen comes into its own at about 18 miles.

In general, there were very mixed results with this full-depletion option – and gradually a more modest model of dietary tinkering evolved. It involves a less arduous training effort about four or five days before the marathon, of about one and a half days of reduced carbohydrate (but not eliminating them), then about two days of loading in the traditional sense. Most of the elite performers use a regime that is closer to this than to the original version, though there are various levels of severity and even at very high level many runners will not be precisely monitoring and quantifying their every mouthful, but will of course be aware of what sort of carb/protein/fat proportions their food contains in the final lead-in to a marathon.

It is maybe worth considering the latest research into this subject by Professor Ron Maughan. He is the World Federation's leading expert on nutrition for endurance and was indeed a very nippy Scottish marathoner in the 1970s. His research shows that the original 'full' version does actually lead to higher levels of muscle glycogen and that a group of subjects tested to exhaustion (for somewhat less than marathon duration) on stationary bikes performed better on this regime. He carefully stops short of stating that this in itself will lead to marathon runners doing quicker races over 26.2 miles by following this regime.

But even with the potential benefits that carbo-loading can bring, do not see it as an elixir that will give you an extra performance bonus beyond what your fitness can provide. Rather, it is a significant piece of icing on the underlying cake (a carb-rich, low-fat cake, of course) – and that cake comprises your training, your taper and, critically, your pace judgement on the day. Nearly all marathoners carbo-load to some degree – can anyone recall a race that offers a pre-race cheese fondue or steak party? – but nearly all still hit the wall because they burn up glycogen far too quickly in the early miles.

Caffeine

There is increasingly robust information that an intake of caffeine can boost long-distance performance because of its effect in enabling the use of fatty acids as an energy source. Tests in 2008 on some non-elite runners showed that all other things being equal, a supplement of 5mg of caffeine per kg of bodyweight led to about a 1.5 per cent increase in performance. That is about 40 seconds in a 10km race or around 3 minutes in a marathon. Based on the caffeine contents of typical drinks, this converts very roughly to about 1–1.5ltr of Coca-Cola; 1ltr of Red Bull or comparable drink; or about three to four 250ml cups of brewed coffee, or about five cups of instant coffee. There are also now a range of gels, bars and capsules that provide the suitable level of caffeine boost. The time frame for ingesting this caffeine is about 30–75 minutes before the event starts. That's quite a lot of coffee or cola to drink in a short time frame and different individuals will have different responses to this sort of regime. It is definitely not advisable to try this for the first time before a big target race, but instead to test it out in a couple of long training runs to judge your overall response to the supplementation.

The side-effects of excess caffeine on a regular basis are well known to many people with no involvement in running. These can include anxiety, dizziness, restlessness and insomnia – all related to the 'buzz' that caffeine gives to the nervous system, so in this case more is definitely not better. You should not take the above-mentioned quantities of caffeine on a continuous basis, because in addition to the adverse health effects you will just minimize the performance boost as your body becomes accustomed to having excess caffeine as its normal state.

Glycogen Intake in Marathons and on Long Training Runs

Looking at the data on your glycogen needs in a marathon versus your body's capacity to store glycogen, the maths indicate that at an even and accurately planned marathon race pace you are about 300–400kcals of glycogen

short of being able to manage to retain some glycogen throughout the race. This equates to three or four gel sachets using the most popular brands, or about four 330ml drinks that have been made up of the same sort of quick-release glycogen compound.

Allowing for the time frame of about 20 minutes from ingesting the carbohydrate to having it available as useable energy in your running muscles, we reach a strategy along the lines of one gel pouch or carbohydrate drink every 4–5km (about 3 miles), starting at about 10–12 miles and depending on where these are actually provided during the race. Or, of course, you can fix the gels to your running kit or slot them into a pocket or customized belt if you prefer to be in control of this factor. As far as replicating this in training, it is sensible to ensure that your digestive system and indeed taste buds can deal with whatever you plan to use on race day, so do check this out. Of course, in training you will not cover the full marathon distance at marathon pace, so you will not exactly replicate the glycogen/fat scenario before race day, but it is definitely advisable to practise your refuelling plan in at least two or three of the longest and hardest training runs.

Beetroot Juice

This is an interesting one because it seems to 'work' in terms of improving endurance, is easily available, natural and has no known long-term adverse effects on health and is therefore legal within all competition rules. In brief, studies at the University of Exeter in 2009 led by Professor Andy Jones, who just happens to be the lead physiologist employed by UK Athletics to work with elite endurance runners, showed that in controlled experiments people could cycle up to 16 per cent longer with a daily half-litre of beetroot juice, and that on a test at high intensity to exhaustion a 2 per cent improvement was noted, on average. Professor Jones stated his 'amazement' at the results, believed to be related to the high nitrate levels in beetroot forming nitric oxide and requiring less oxygen to be taken in to maintain a given level of aerobic effort. He made the caveat that the tests were done using cycling rather than running and the subjects were not elite athletes.

It is notable that after an initial surge in media interest and beetroot juice talk and intake in the running community, it is no longer centre-stage. For an elite athlete, 2 per cent is a big gain, especially if it is risk-free, guaranteed and can be gained in such a simple process as a pint of vegetable juice.

On the other hand, it would be very hard for a distance runner making a 2 per cent improvement in real competition performance (as opposed to a lab test) to isolate the progression to just one factor such as beetroot juice. That said, in autumn 2011 two Canadian elite marathoners both ran notable PBs in Toronto, securing selection for the 2012 Olympics. One took a pint (half-litre) of beetroot juice with his pre-race meal, the other took the same amount about two days before the race (having had stomach problems with drinking it too close to the race time). There is no evidence that longer-term beetroot juice intake produces any further aerobic gains so, thankfully, runners need not contemplate a lifetime of discharging dark purple urine. At the time of writing, it is a case of 'watch this space' or, more specifically, check out what is probably the first time a Suffolk vegetable farm has been so closely linked to high-performance sports science.

For further information, please see Further Reading.

KEY POINTS

- Understand the basics, but do not obsess or overestimate the significance.
- Try to follow the guidelines relating to the refuelling window to aid recovery.
- Female runners in particular should be aware of ferretin levels.
- The carbohydrate loading (possibly preceded by mild depletion) option should have benefit in marathons if the runner handles marathon pace sensibly.
- Use longer training runs to practise glycogen and fluid replacement strategies and avoid experimenting in key races.
- Consider experimenting with a palatable form of beetroot juice – it may be a 'one per center'.

CHAPTER 10

INJURY FACTORS

'Search for the Silver Line Message'.

John Buchanan,
Australian National Cricket Coach

Overview of Overuse Injuries

Injuries are an inevitable part of running for most people. But before looking at the physical factors, it is worth a brief analysis of the mental side of sports injuries, as this has generated some sports science research in its own right. An injured runner is inevitably a less content person than an uninjured runner and how we treat injuries will affect both our future running and, at least in the short term, our state of mind, so it is worth trying to make the most of whatever obstacles we have to deal with. Leaving aside elite professionals where a severe injury can threaten their financial livelihood, committed amateur runners can place great store by their running, which is often linked to social networks, self-esteem, weight management and stress relief, so without our regular training 'dose' we lose much more than just the physiological effect of the missed training sessions.

To show the prevalence of running injuries, the following data was provided from over 200 runners in a London survey. The respondents represented a typical cross-section of long-distance runners, with over 95 per cent being in the twenty-five to fifty-five age group; 53 per cent running between

Prevalence of Running Injuries in a London Survey

Condition	Percentage Affected in Last Month	Perentage Affected over Running Career
Knee pain	19	69
Iliotibial band syndrome	8	58
Shin splints	3	42
Hip pain	13	40
Achilles tendonosis	6	36
Plantar fasciitis	3	30
Stress fracture	2	20
Piriformis syndrome	5	18
Other	9	47

20–40 miles per week; 14 per cent running between 40–60 miles weekly; 45 per cent with less than five years' running history; and 27 per cent with between five to ten years' running on the clock. Clearly, the table opposite is a summary, with no measurement of the injuries' severity and in some cases, such as 'knee pain', wrapping up a range of complex symptoms into a generalized category.

If one takes a pragmatic view of these stats – or cynical view, maybe – the percentages in the final column will inevitably rise as the runners' number of years in the sport increases. Suffice to say that sports medicine providers seeking to develop their understanding of running injuries are, quite reasonably, balancing the profession's Hippocratic ideals with good business sense.

Whilst occasional impact or direct injuries can affect endurance runners – famous examples include Paula Radcliffe injuring a knee whilst signing her wedding invitations and Steve Ovett slamming his knee into some church railings whilst training – the vast majority of distance-running injuries are through overuse. So, frustratingly, the running movement that builds up your fitness is the same running movement that may injure you.

Bear in mind that 'overuse' is a deliberately generic word that in running injury terms can simply mean 'too much' in the widest sense. Too much mileage per se, of course, but it can also include any of the following causes:

- too much running on pavement or tarmac;
- too much running in inadequate shoes;
- too rapid an increase in the volume of training;
- too rapid an increase in the intensity of training, even if the volume has stayed the same;
- too sudden a change in the training regime, whether related to the running

and/or non-running elements of the training programme;
- too much uphill or downhill running;
- too much running on an uneven road camber;
- too much training on an inadequately nourished or dehydrated body;
- too much training on a sleep-deprived body;
- too much running for the body's particular state of biomechanics.

That's a lot of factors, so it is no wonder that so many runners suffer some sort of injury at some point. It does, however, back up the overarching philosophy of making training progress gradually rather than suddenly.

Working with Medical Advice

If we exclude degenerative conditions such as advanced osteoarthritis and trauma injuries that may permanently damage your musculoskeletal structure, then there really should be very, very few injuries that are somehow 'caused' by running that should need to end your running career. You may need to do extensive rehab exercises; you may eventually need to consider the benefits of minor surgery; you may need to be very careful about surfaces, very long distances, frequency of running, or footwear; but one way or another there should be a source of treatment that keeps you as a regular endurance runner.

The word 'conditioning' has just as wide a coverage and for distance running we can maybe think of it in modern management speak as meaning 'fit for purpose'. There are elite runners whose marathon preparation may include up to 130 miles weekly on the roads and if they can sustain this without any of the above factors taking a toll then one

Most Common Running Injuries

Injury Type	Symptoms	Typical Causes	Possible Treatments
Achilles tendonosis (inaccurately often described as 'tendonitis')	Pain on and around the Achilles heel area, particularly on rising in the morning and at the beginning of a run	Tight calf muscles, over pronation and overzealous increase in hill training or faster running	Calf raises to increase strength and mobility – rigorous progressive programme advised. Massage
Iliotibial band syndrome (ITBS)	Sharp pain on the outer side of the knee as a result of the tendon becoming inflamed	Any combination of the overuse factors, particularly downhill running, pronation or tight lower and big hip flexors	Increase flexibility of tight areas. Massage of ITB including self-massage with tennis ball or foam roller. Can be a very insidious problem to get rid of
Piriformis syndrome	Deep pain in buttock area may be linked with painful stabbing feeling down hamstring if sciatic nerve compressed	Any weakness or imbalance around major muscle groups in lower back; glutes; hip flexors or abductors or hamstrings	Massage affected area and surrounds; if piriformis is in spasm, can be quickly released by external massage. Also use tennis or golf ball as self-massage to stave off tightness
Plantar fasciitis	Acute pain under front and middle part of foot, particularly on rising in morning. Caused by inflammation of the plantar fascia tendon	Combination of overuse factors, plus weak foot muscles or high arches	Ice or contrast bathing (alternate hot and cold water for 5–10 minute spells). Self-massage with golf or tennis ball. 'Night boot' also particularly useful to stretch out the plantar fascia and reduce pain in 7–14 days
Runner's knee (patellofemoral pain syndrome)	Stabbing deep pain around kneepcap, particularly going downhill or downstairs	Poor tracking of knee as it moves, related to imbalance or weakness in surrounding muscles and tendons, particularly vastus medials, the inner quadriceps. Flat feet or weak pelvic area	Strengthening relevant areas by single leg squats and step ups onto chair or step
Sciatica	Acute stabbing pain anywhere from the lower back down through the glutes, hamstrings and the calf	Any inflammation or displacement of the third, fourth or fifth lumbar vertebrae or of the first sacral vertebra (lower back, broadly), which presses on the sciatic nerve	Combination of rest, anti-inflammatory treatment and physio/massage to alleviate the area causing the pain (normally not the prime site of the pain). Also try – with care and correct technique – nerve stretches; the Slump for the lower back, glutes and hamstrings, and Point and Flex for where the nerve passes through the calf to the Achilles

Shin splints	Pain around the inner lower leg/shin. Can become acute quickly, but can also disappear quickly after rest in early stages	Combination of overuse factors cause inflammation of the medial tibia where the muscle meets the bone	Massage the affected area, plus ice, plus anti-inflammatory gel. Avoid hard surfaces, overused trainers and downhills while recovering. Also strengthen calf and shin muscles
Stress fractures	Specific sharp pain, most commonly in metatarsals (feet and toes) and in shin. Also there is now a lower-level 'stress reaction', in layman's terms a halfway house that needs to be rested for a much shorter timescale to prevent it becoming a stress fracture	Combination of overuse factors. Rarely show up on an X-ray, so an X-ray is not at all conclusive	The recovery period seems in nearly all cases to be close to six weeks and 'testing' the injury any earlier is very likely to cause a relapse. Avoid weight-bearing training during rehab period

way or another they have become adequately conditioned to do so.

The runner's perception of the quality of their medical adviser is key in the recovery process and is linked to their diligence in following the recommended rehab programme. So, just as with your running, do set some goals and structure your non-running recovery process. If your practitioner is as committed to eliminating and preventing the injury's recurrence as you are likely to be, there may be a regular and precise set of exercises and drills that you are advised to do. Two or three sessions per day is not uncommon from sports medicine specialists, maybe spending up to 40 or 50 minutes daily building up the conditioning needed to reduce the prospects of the injury recurring. This has the added benefit that mentally you will still have that structure and commitment to a training plan, albeit that it won't involve belting round your most scenic training routes.

When you decide that an injury does need some medical diagnosis and advice, take a pen and paper to your first appointment (which may be your only appointment if you are lucky) and ask your specialist all of the following, then note down and act upon the replies:

- What caused the injury?
- What exactly should I do to prevent the injury recurring?
- How often should I do the rehab exercises and how long should I continue to do them for?
- How long should I cease running for?
- When I start running, how should I build up the running duration and frequency?
- What cross-training options can I pursue in the meantime?
- Can I do these cross-training options with the same intensity as my running?

Your practitioner may not be able to provide all of the answers, but it's definitely worth asking. Bear in mind that the healing process may vary in duration and that a second or in some case third appointment may also be recommended. It is an annoying scenario for any runner to be in – not only are you unable to run, but you are incurring extra expense and probably spending what would be training or leisure time in travelling to appointments and doing the recommended rehab. Do follow the rehab advice precisely as recommended, however time-consuming and boring it may be. If you don't, you are more likely to be making additional visits if the injury recurs.

There is a major link between the conditioning of a runner, their biomechanics and their incidence of injury. So if you find that you increase your average mileage from say 30 to 40 miles over two months and become injured in doing so, on the one hand it may well be that the increased mileage partly caused the injury. On the other hand, don't take this to mean that you will repeatedly become injured when you run 40 miles weekly. It should be a matter of increasing the strength/strength-endurance qualities of whatever caused the injury (quite often more than one factor is involved), so that you can in future withstand a higher training load, if that is how you wish to progress.

The often quoted guideline of avoiding mileage increases of more than 10 per cent per week has its general uses, but it does not acknowledge that each runner will have an injury threshold, which will vary as their robustness increases or decreases, so if you are having recurring injuries keep a tab on how your mileage has evolved and look for indicators of what may be your cut-off point. Also bear in mind that if the increased training creates an injury after months of pain-free running, the degree of 'fault' that needs remedying is probably not that vast because it has managed to get you through several months of decent training at a slightly lower level.

The consensus amongst sports coaches through recent decades is that sports medi-

KEY POINTS

- Persevere with medically advised rehab exercises when injury strikes.
- Virtually all overuse injuries can be treated to enable a return to regular running.
- Be as methodical in your approach to injury treatment as you are to other parts of your training and racing.
- Shoe manufacturers' recommendations on a shoe's optimum mileage are rooted in science as well as marketing practices.
- Use your training logs to evaluate what may be a breaking point in your injury-avoidance plans.

cine is becoming ever more widely understood and practised, and indeed medical students now have the option of pursuing sports medicine as their specialism at a much earlier stage in their careers than used to be feasible. Not surprisingly, many sports doctors are or were committed sports players, so will share the runner's mindset about being motivated to get back into training as soon as possible.

There's no escaping the fact that if you wish to be treated quickly, taking the private medicine route will invariably offer a speedier response than using National Health Service provisions, and experience suggests that you may indeed receive a longer appointment slot for a more holistic diagnosis. However, there are sports medical practitioners who split their time between public and private systems, so there is not an assumption that you won't be offered a high level of technical expertise through the NHS.

Of course, the Internet also enables us to take the riskier route of becoming our own physician by typing our symptoms into a search engine and seeing what is the best match of diagnosis. The great pluses of this 'system' are that it is free, easy to access and does not require you to sit in a doctor's waiting room flicking absently through glossy magazines. The obvious downside is that it offers less than 100 per cent reliability.

The large majority of all running injuries will fall within the issues described in outline in the accompanying table. You should also be aware of the anatomical links throughout your body, which mean that although you may experience pain at a particular place, the root cause of the problem may well be somewhere else in the body. Also, once you carry on running with a low-level injury, the small changes in movement you are likely to make to 'nurse' the injury's site will, multiplied by the thousands of strides you will take, be likely to trigger compensatory problems elsewhere.

For further information, see the Further Reading section.

RACE SELECTIONS

Because this book is targeted at runners already with some grounding in the sport, there seems little benefit in highlighting the major domestic and international races that are known even by non-runners, let alone established endurance athletes. So the likes of the Great North Run, the Virgin London Marathon and the other global major marathons such as New York, Berlin and Paris will no doubt already be on people's radars and need no further promotion here. What is shown below is a list of options, domestic and international, that you may wish to consider to combine some weekend city-hopping with a good-quality well-organized distance race. It goes nowhere near to being a thorough race calendar, but from the author's experience and feedback from runners it offers some hidden gems.

The overseas races are all within Europe. Of course, there are numerous good-quality events all over the planet, but by and large the logistics of travel, time-zone changes and of course long-haul air fares mean that in practice most running trips beyond British shores by British runners are within Europe. The races are listed in calendar order so that readers can more readily see what fits into their own domestic circumstances over a given year.

Several of the main European marathons are timetabled with a half-marathon in the same city between four and twelve weeks beforehand. These may also be worth exploring, particularly if organized by the same qual-

ity assured team that organizes the city's marathon.

If you haven't raced abroad before, do not assume that everything in an overseas race is organized exactly as one would expect in the UK. Check out aspects like the start and finish areas; transport from your accommodation to the start area, particularly if there are any changes or restrictions on race day; refreshments on the course; whether the start zone is divided up by predicted finish time or is a free-for-all. Also check that your hotel will provide breakfast early enough for your normal race-day meal – and remember that 6 o'clock on Sunday morning is not the busiest time for European city life. If in doubt, buy suitable food and drink the previous day. If there are any dietary 'must haves' that are your particular nutritional comfort blanket, maybe take them as part of your luggage.

You should minimize risk and take your racing shoes in your hand luggage; you will have a physically and emotionally fraught weekend if you tackle the Reykjavik marathon while your favourite snugly fitting racing shoes are waiting unclaimed at Moscow airport.

The dates below are correct as at autumn 2011. Most races, once established, tend to use the same weekend each year, but changes may occasionally occur.

The more regularly you race, the more you may need to accept that you won't set a PB each time, particularly if you have set your best time on a flat course, in ideal weather, with a sensible taper and good pace judgement on

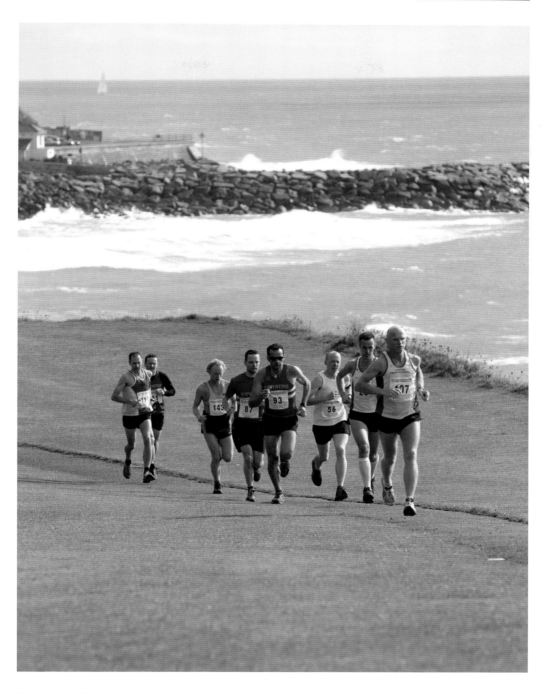

Scenic races often mean tough climbs.

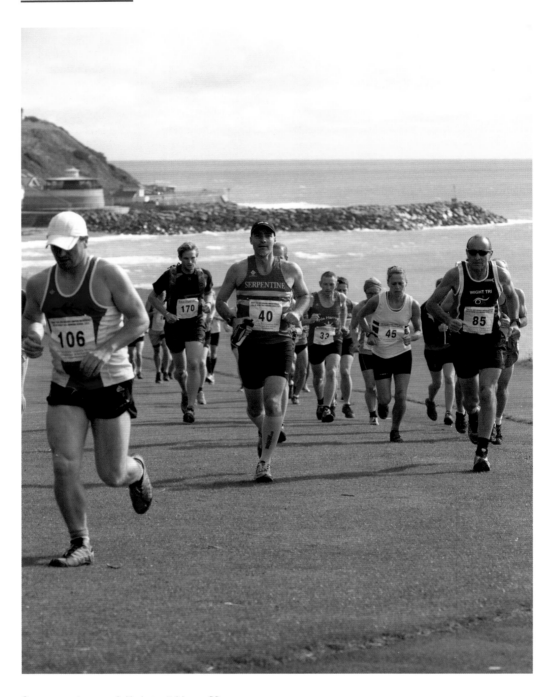

Some races just aren't likely to yield new PBs.

the day. So don't worry about taking in some undulating races. Be aware that it often seems that race directors have taken their understanding of words like 'flat', 'mildly undulating', 'gentle gradient' from how a Himalayan sherpa might perceive them.

The most extensive link for international quality-assured marathons and half-marathons is AIMS (Association of International Marathons: www.aimsworldrunning.org), which has links to each individual event website.

January
- Helsby Half-Marathon, Cheshire – useful option in a month with few other longer race options. www.helsbyrunningclub.org.uk

February
- Great Bentley Half-Marathon – fast course in Essex. www.gbrc.org.uk
- Seville Marathon – very flat and fast, well organized and usually offers good running weather. www.imd.sevilla.org/maraton/EN

March
- Rhayader 20 miles – wonderful scenic race in the Elan Valley, useful prep for April marathons if you don't go right to your limit. Hilly first 5 miles, then mainly flattish. www.rhayaderac.org.uk/20mile.htm
- Wilmslow Half-Marathon – usually one of the key build-up races for spring marathons. www.wilmslowhalf.org.uk

April
- Bungay Black Dog Marathon and Half-Marathon – scenic and low-key, but well-established races in rural Suffolk. Nice break for city dwellers and London Marathon 'rejects'. www.bungayblackdogrunningclub.co.uk/marathon

May
- Sunderland Marathon of the North – brand new event starting 2012. Steve Cram is Event Director and that should ensure the event is of a high standard. www.marathonofthenorth.co.uk
- Riga Marathon mid to late May, fast-growing Baltic option pitched just before warmer weather likely to be a factor. www.nordearigasmaratons.lv/en

June
- Stockholm Marathon – scenic course through beautiful waterside city. Can be warmer than ideal and post-race beers not the cheapest. www.stockholmmarathon.se
- North Downs 30km – suitable for those targeting early autumn marathons. Receives incredibly high satisfaction ratings. www.isteadandifield.org.uk
- Tromsø midnight sun marathon – unique North Polar region race, actually on a fast course. Two flights needed to arrive there from UK. www.msm.no

July
- High Wycombe Half-Marathon – long established race in Bucks, one major climb, one big descent, but otherwise mainly flat. www.handycrossrunners.co.uk

August
- Reykjavik Marathon, Iceland – the only mainstream city marathon in Europe in summer, making the most of Iceland's climate. www.marathon.is/reykjavik-marathon
- Burnham Beeches Half-Marathon – good, scenic but tough hilly option for those doing early autumn marathons. The local beeches along much of the course provide shadow on hotter days. www.burnhamjoggers.org.uk

October

- Cabbage Patch 10 Miles, Twickenham, London – well-known fast course, also used as a build-up towards late autumn marathons. Contrary to first impressions, the prize winners do receive handy prizes in addition to the outsize cabbages. www.cabbagepatch10.com
- Ridgeway Run – 15km in Tring, Herts. Mixed terrain with fantastic views of the Chilterns. Useful test build-up to a November target race. www.tringrunningclub.org.uk
- Eindhoven Marathon – a week before Amsterdam, is every bit as flat, fast and well-organized as its more famous Dutch counterpart. www.marathoneindhoven.nl
- Abingdon Marathon – fast and flat, entry limit of 1,100 is filled months in advance, even before the London Marathon has taken place. www.abingdonmarathon.org.uk
- Istanbul Eurasia Marathon – uniquely, the race covers two continents with stunning views across the Bosphorus Straits that divide Europe from Asia. Some early climbs, but largely flat after 15km. www.istanbulmarathon.org

November

- San Sebastiàn Marathon – flat, well-organized course in the fascinating Basque region of Spain, in one of its most attractive cities. www.maratondonostia.com
- Florence Marathon – fast and well organized, another cultural centre building a sizeable international event. www.firenzemarathon.it
- Valencia Marathon – fastest times recorded in Spain, another well-reputed event in an interesting and developing city; date has recently been changed from February. www.maratondivinapastoravalencia.com

December

- Pisa Marathon – last sizeable European city marathon before Christmas period. www.pisamarathon.it
- Seville Half-Marathon – mid December. Flat and fast and a great escape from pre-Christmas routines, at a time when few such races are held in the UK. www.rfea.es/calendario/ruta

FURTHER READING

Bean, Anita, *Complete Guide to Sports Nutrition 6th Edition* (London: A & C Black)

Griffin, Jane, *Food for Sport: Eat Well, Perform Better* (Ramsbury: The Crowood Press)

Grisogono, Vivian, *Running Fitness and Injuries* (London: John Murray)

Maughan, Ron J., *Food, Nutrition and Sports Performance II* (Oxford: Routledge)

Noakes, Tim, *Lore of Running – Human Kinetics* (Oxford: OUP)

Norris, Christopher, *The Complete Guide to Stretching* (Complete Guides)

Peterson, Lars and Renstrom, Per, *Sports Injuries – Their Prevention and Treatment* (Oxford: Martin Dunitz)

Spedding, Charlie, *From Last to First* (London: Aurum Press)

Stear, Samantha, *Fuelling Fitness for Sports Performance* (London: British Olympic Association)

Tulloh, Bruce, *Running over 40,50,60,70…* (Tulloh Books)

INDEX